Prevention Science & Targeted Methods for HIV/STI Research with Black Sexual Minority Men

Derek T. Dangerfield II

Prevention Science & Targeted Methods for HIV/STI Research with Black Sexual Minority Men

Springer

Derek T. Dangerfield II
Department of Prevention and Community Health
George Washington University,
Milken Institute School of Public Health
Washington, DC, USA

ISBN 978-3-031-85132-2 ISBN 978-3-031-85130-8 (eBook)
https://doi.org/10.1007/978-3-031-85130-8

This Springer imprint is published by the registered company Springer Nature Switzerland AG
The registered company address is: Gewerbestrasse 11, 6330 Cham, Switzerland

Foreword

The health and well-being of Black gay, bisexual, and other Black sexual minority men has been a vital yet challenging area of research, education, and practice. This community has borne a markedly disproportionate burden of HIV and other sexually transmitted infections while having, on an individual level, lower sexual risks for these infections than other US sexual minority men. This paradox has brought to the fore the essential realities of the social determinants of health for these men and has highlighted the importance of the many intersectional challenges they have faced in seeking to live healthy sexual and romantic lives. These intersecting barriers include the stigma and discrimination associated with racial and sexual minority status, including anti-Black racism, unfair housing, restricted employment opportunities, and aggressive policing in the USA. Taken together, these realities demand engaged and community-based efforts to address these complex interactions. And they demand that Black resilience, joy, and community strengths be part of intervention strategies. This is not easy work. And so, it makes it all the more valuable for those in the field, and for affected communities, to have Dr. Derek T, Dangerfield II as a resource and guide.

Dr. Dangerfield is an experienced prevention scientist who has dedicated his career to the well-being of Black sexual minority men. His new book *Prevention Science and Targeted Methods for HIV/STI Research with Black Sexual Minority Men* is a readable yet technically solid tool for investigators, providers, learners, and community members who seek to do better for the men they serve. This is a work of both heart and head, where Dangerfield's deep concern for his community shines as brightly as his expertise as a leader in HIV prevention research. It is practical, is grounded in theory, and takes a "hands-on" approach to doing this vital work that will benefit many. I, for one, am grateful to Dr. Dangerfield for taking this on, and for producing such a timely and helpful text for the field.

Duke Global Health Institute,

Durham, NC, USA Chris Beyrer

Preface

Sexual health, as defined by global health organizations, extends beyond the absence of disease and includes access to comprehensive information, supportive environments, and the ability to engage in pleasurable, safe, and consensual sexual experiences. The intersection of sexual health inequalities and the evolving landscape of prevention science necessitates a renewed and targeted focus on populations that are disproportionately impacted by HIV and STIs. Among these, Black gay, bisexual, and other Black sexual minority men (SMM) remain at the forefront, facing unique challenges that require effective, culturally competent, and scientifically robust interventions. For Black SMM, sexual health is often affected by social inequalities, stigmas, and health beliefs that perpetuate differences in outcomes. The persistent negative sexual health outcomes within the community, including HIV and STIs, underscores the urgency for contemporary approaches that not only address risks but also provide a comprehensive understanding of the social, behavioral, and cultural factors that amplify vulnerability. Addressing sexual health disparities and inequities requires intentional focus and strategies that incorporate community engagement, policy reform, and education initiatives to build trust and ensure relevant approaches. This handbook, *Prevention Science and Targeted Methods for HIV/STI Research with Black SMM*, emerges as both a response to and a roadmap for addressing the crucial needs of this highly vulnerable and misunderstood community.

This book builds on a decade of targeted research and practice with Black SMM throughout the USA, offering a compendium of frameworks, techniques, and strategies to enhance prevention science. It integrates advances in biomedical, behavioral, and structural interventions, highlighting their usefulness as both independent and complementary approaches. From groundbreaking developments in pre-exposure prophylaxis (PrEP) and treatment as prevention (TasP) to the emergence of digital health tools and peer-based initiatives, this handbook underscores the importance of leveraging traditional prevention methods with innovations targeting the unique vulnerabilities of US Black SMM. The chapters are structured to guide readers through a comprehensive examination of sexual health research and intervention design. Each chapter addresses key aspects of prevention science, from epidemiological overviews to advanced methodologies for participant engagement and intervention delivery. The focus is not merely on identifying nuanced challenges, but also on proposing actionable solutions rooted in empirical evidence and cultural responsiveness.

A unique aspect of this handbook is its shifted focus from risk and deficit frameworks towards more empowerment models that promote holistic well-being. This shift is particularly vital for Black SMM, whose sexual health narratives have often been shaped by stigma and deficit-focused discourse. Another key aspect of this handbook includes a particular focus on research ethics, which are often overlooked or insufficiently addressed in studies involving marginalized populations. Considering the role of research ethics helps ensure that research practices not only protect the rights and dignity of participants but also actively work to build trust within the community. This ethical commitment includes addressing power dynamics between researchers and participants, ensuring informed consent processes are transparent and culturally sensitive, and fostering collaborations that prioritize the voices and needs of Black SMM. The handbook seeks to redefine the relationship between researchers and communities (including community members as researchers) and lay the groundwork for interventions that are both impactful and equitable.

This handbook can serve as both a resource and an inspiration for scientists, clinicians, and public health practitioners. It provides practical tools and strategies while fostering a deeper understanding of the sociocultural dynamics influencing health behaviors and outcomes among Black SMM. This handbook aims to empower stakeholders with evidence-based strategies and innovative approaches to confront these challenges, fostering a path toward equitable health outcomes. Furthermore, it underscores the importance of integrating community voices and lived experiences to ensure interventions resonate authentically and effectively with those they aim to serve. Whether you are an emerging prevention scientist or a seasoned expert, the insights presented herein will equip you to design and implement interventions that are comprehensive, impactful, and transformative.

Navigating the intricate terrain of sexual health requires a unified and unwavering commitment to change. This handbook serves as a clarion call for action, urging stakeholders to critically examine the multifaceted factors driving inequities and to foster collaboration across disciplines. The challenge to address these disparities demands sustained dedication to research, innovative intervention strategies, and the pursuit of health equity. Centering the voices and lived experiences of Black SMM remains paramount, ensuring that their needs, perspectives, and strengths guide every step of the process. This focus aims to create a future where sexual health is recognized as a fundamental right accessible to all, transcending privilege and systemic barriers. By working collectively, prevention scientists, clinicians, policymakers, and community advocates can advance the field of prevention science and forge a more inclusive, just, and equitable healthcare landscape.

Washington, DC Derek T. Dangerfield II

Competing Interests The author has no competing interests to declare that are relevant to the content of this manuscript.

Competing Interests The author has no competing interests to declare that are relevant to the content of this manuscript.

Introduction to Sexual Health, HIV/STI Epidemiology, and the Prevention Science Landscape

Sexual Health Overview

According to the World Health Organization (WHO), sexual health focuses on the consequences of unprotected sexual activity, access to comprehensive, high-quality information and healthcare, and living in an environment that promotes sexual health (WHO, 2006, 2024). Sexual health also focuses on ensuring that sexual experiences are pleasurable, safe, and free from coercion, discrimination, and violence (Office of the Surgeon General (US) & Office of Population Affairs (US), 2001; WHO, 2024). HIV/STI prevention researchers are increasingly calling for more gain-frame discourse (Poteat & Logie, 2022), which focuses on the positive outcomes of engaging in prevention behaviors rather than emphasizing the negative consequences of not doing so. Data show that emphasizing the benefits of condom use or regular HIV testing increases the likelihood that people engage in these prevention behaviors (Hull, 2020; Bannon & Schwartz, 2020), suggesting that gain-framed sexual health messages could be effective for promoting health behaviors. These perspectives align with "sex-positive epidemiology," which incorporates pleasure, satisfaction, and well-being into research alongside traditional sexual health outcomes such as STIs (Bond & Ford, 2024). Sex-positive frameworks can also be considered to be grounded in traditional behavioral science theories that suggest that people are more likely to engage in prevention behaviors when they perceive (and understand) the benefits of those actions (Fishbein & Yzer, 2003; Rosenstock, 1974a). Advocates have called for an even more holistic view of sexual health that includes a focus on other socioecological factors such as racism and stigma to reflect a broader, more comprehensive approach to understanding and addressing sexual health issues for minority populations (Bowleg et al., 2022; Coleman et al., 2016; Dean & Fenton, 2010; Sharpe et al., 2011). This broader view of sexual health is essential for addressing the persistent and significant impact of HIV and STIs on affected minority populations.

The Significance of HIV and STIs

HIV and other STIs remain a significant public health threat. HIV has profound negative impacts on both individuals and communities, affecting health, social dynamics, and economic stability. HIV attacks the immune system, targeting CD4 cells (or T cells), which are crucial for fighting infections in the body. Without effective and consistent treatment, HIV can lead to AIDS, severely compromising the immune system and increasing individual susceptibility to opportunistic infections, certain cancers, and ultimately, premature mortality. Living with HIV can increase exposure to stigma and discrimination, and also affect mental health issues such as stress, depression, anxiety, and hopelessness, especially among Black gay, bisexual, and other Black sexual minority men (SMM) who already experience background prejudice, discrimination, and marginalization in society.

Similarly, STIs can also cause severe health issues (Craib et al., 1995; Deguchi et al., 2012; Solomon et al., 2014; Unemo & Jensen, 2017). For example, untreated STIs can cause paralysis and blindness (via syphilis and gonorrhea), infertility (via gonorrhea and chlamydia), and several forms of cancer (via human papillomavirus) (Etheridge et al., 2019; Lin et al., 2017; Piketty et al., 2008). Untreated STIs also facilitate multidrug-resistant bacteria for which treatments are failing. The throat particularly facilitates gonococcal antimicrobial resistance partly due to inadequate screening and treatment adherence (Deguchi et al., 2012; Gaspari et al., 2019). Most extragenital (pharyngeal and rectal) STIs can be asymptomatic and are not always treated thoroughly partly because clinicians do not routinely screen their patients for them (Deguchi et al., 2012; Patton et al., 2014; Watson et al., 2022). Moreover, STIs exacerbate HIV acquisition and transmission risk. Gonorrhea, chlamydia, syphilis, herpes simplex virus type 2, and monkeypox create lesions that increase inflammatory immune cells in the body and facilitate HIV acquisition (Fleming & Wasserheit, 1999; Li et al., 2016; Mayer & Venkatesh, 2011; Rottingen et al., 2001). Syphilis and rectal gonorrhea are independently associated with HIV acquisition (Craib et al., 1995; Solomon et al., 2014). Data show that 7.8%–12.2% of HIV incidence among Black SMM is attributable to chlamydia and gonorrhea alone (Chesson et al., 2021). STIs increase the risk of both HIV and STI transmission among people living with HIV (Fleming & Wasserheit, 1999; Wasserheit, 1992). Therefore, the downstream effects of prevalent and undertreated STIs indicate a significant public health problem.

Economically, HIV and STIs pose a substantial burden on both individuals and society. The cost of lifelong antiretroviral therapy (ART) for HIV treatment is substantial but is also required to manage the virus over the life course. The need for continuous medical care can strain public health systems particularly in low-resource settings because people living with HIV require sustained resource allocation, increasing financial burdens and demanding consistently high levels of healthcare workforce engagement to manage their care (Chesson et al., 2021; Schackman et al., 2015). Since HIV disproportionately affects marginalized, minority communities, demographic differences in incidence rates can exacerbate existing social inequities. The economic impact of HIV/STIs also includes lost productivity due to illness and premature death, which affects the economic stability of families, communities, and society. Comprehensive strategies to address these impacts are essential to improving the quality of life for populations that are affected by HIV/STIs to mitigate the broader social consequences of infectious disease epidemiology.

HIV/STIs Among Black Sexual Minority Men

US HIV/STI epidemiology highlights a crucial need to focus prevention efforts on Black SMM. From 2000 to 2017, HIV incidence remained unchanged among Black SMM generally and increased by 42% for those aged 25–34 (Centers for Disease Control and Prevention, 2020; Jeffries IV et al., 2020). In 2019, Black SMM accounted for 37% of new diagnoses among gay and bisexual men (CDC, 2020). The CDC acknowledged that between 2010 and 2019, no progress was made in reducing disparities in HIV incidence for Black gay and bisexual men (Pitasi, 2021). Increased focus has been directed toward young Black SMM in particular, for whom HIV rates are most disproportionate compared to all other US SMM groups (CDC, 2020; Koblin et al., 2013). Effective HIV prevention and treatment strategies to address the persistent disparities and reduce the disproportionate impact of HIV on Black SMM are still needed.

For people living with HIV, retention in care, treatment adherence, and viral suppression are key to eliminating HIV transmission risk because maintaining an undetectable viral load prevents the virus from being transmitted to others (Eisinger et al., 2019). However, only 55% of Black SMM living with HIV maintain their care, only 58% have 100% daily treatment adherence, and of those, only 62% are virally suppressed or undetectable (CDC, 2020). Black SMM are less likely than any other gay/bisexual men living with HIV to be retained in care, adhere to treatment, or achieve viral suppression (Hoots et al., 2017; Sullivan et al., 2021). Concurrently, pre-exposure prophylaxis (PrEP) use among HIV-negative gay/bisexual men also remains lowest for Black SMM and increases their vulnerability to acquiring HIV from individuals who are not virally suppressed (Bonett et al., 2021; Quinn et al., 2018; Shover et al., 2018; Volk et al., 2015). Therefore, the combination of low viral suppression and low PrEP use among Black SMM will perpetuate community HIV transmission.

Surveillance data also continue to show that gonorrhea, syphilis, and chlamydia have reached an all-time high for Black SMM (Centers for Disease Control and Prevention, 2016; Scott-Sheldon & Chan, 2020; Workowski, 2021). Other STIs such as Mpox and mycoplasma genitalium are also increasing and resisting treatment (Machalek et al., 2020; Unemo & Jensen, 2017). Syphilis and pharyngeal gonorrhea incidence for Black SMM is respectively 4.6 and 2 times as high as white SMM (CDC, 2017; Mustanski et al., 2017). Rectal STIs among SMM are also highest for Black men (Johnson Jones et al., 2019; Mustanski et al., 2017). One study found that a prior gonorrhea or chlamydia infection increased the likelihood of a future STI among Black SMM 15-fold (Burns et al., 2020). Repeated STIs are also prevalent among those using PrEP for HIV prevention (Wood & Guthrie, 2022; Zeggagh et al., 2022). Repeated STIs exponentially increase the risks for negative mental health outcomes, HIV transmission (among individuals who are not using PrEP), and treatment resistance (Bernstein et al., 2010). Notably, evidence of the increased HIV and STI risk among Black SMM has been unremitting for 20 years, underscoring the sexual health disparities among gay and bisexual men, including an unrefuted estimated 50% lifetime HIV risk for Black SMM (Hess et al., 2017; Maulsby et al., 2013; Millett et al., 2006, 2012; Sullivan et al., 2021).

Explaining Sexual Health Disparities

Conventional risk behaviors such as condomless anal intercourse do not explain the HIV disparities between Black SMM and other gay and bisexual men. Several systematic reviews and meta-analyses have highlighted that Black SMM are more likely than others to report any prevention behavior against HIV infection, including condom use, HIV testing, fewer sex partners, and less drug use before or during sex (Maulsby et al., 2013; Millett et al., 2012; Sullivan et al., 2015). Instead, socioecological factors such as socioeconomic status, healthcare access, stigma, and discrimination from clinicians remain barriers that increase disease vulnerability for Black SMM. The COVID-19 pandemic further complicated the sexual health landscape and underscored existing inequities in healthcare, disproportionately affecting marginalized communities who already face barriers. These barriers limit access to and use of HIV prevention and treatment services, sustaining health disparities even though individuals might be more engaged in protective behaviors than others. Addressing these socioecological factors is crucial for developing effective interventions and ensuring equitable health outcomes for Black SMM. Prevention scientists and clinicians must understand these background and contemporary contexts of disease epidemiology to design targeted, multifaceted interventions that address the unique vulnerability among Black SMM.

The Current Sexual Health Prevention Science Landscape

Prevention science promotes sexual health using four key activities: (1) identifying the public health problem; (2) identifying risk and protective factors; (3) designing and testing interventions; and (4) implementing effective strategies (interventions). Prevention science also includes involving communities in their own health behaviors and targeting interventions to their specific needs (Office of the Surgeon General (US) & Office of Population Affairs (US), 2001). Prevention science plays a crucial role in sexual health promotion by designing and implementing evidence-based strategies that prevent negative outcomes including HIV/STIs and other sexual health issues to improve overall health and quality of life.

Over the past 35 years, the prevention science field has made significant advances that have improved the understanding of culture, sexuality, and health, even among Black SMM. For example, large-scale surveys of sexual behavior that were initiated in the 1980s due to the emergence of the HIV epidemic were initially politically controversial but have since gained acceptance globally. Longitudinal studies of minority communities have also become more prevalent, offering valuable data on changes in sexual behavior and health over time. Additionally, sampling strategies, survey question standardization, and computer-assisted data collection methods have increasingly enhanced data quality. Biological measures such as the presence of STIs and drug concentrations have also been increasingly integrated into behavioral studies. Qualitative research methods have also increasingly been integrated alongside quantitative surveys to obtain deeper insights into the experiences, behaviors, and attitudes of marginalized communities. Technological advances such as mobile health applications have improved real-time data collection and intervention delivery. Moreover, collaborative efforts between researchers, public health practitioners, and community organizations have also strengthened team science and the relevance and application of research findings. All of these advancements have allowed researchers to obtain a more comprehensive understanding of sexual health and behavior, facilitating the design of more effective community health interventions. Integrating this range of approaches into public health frameworks is crucial for sustaining HIV/STI prevention efforts, reducing sexual health disparities, and promoting health equity.

Biomedical Interventions

Biomedical interventions refer to medical, technological, and pharmacological methods to prevent disease acquisition and transmission and have revolutionized the HIV/STI prevention landscape. One of the most notable advancements is PrEP, which initially involved a once-daily oral medication to prevent disease acquisition among HIV-negative individuals. Studies have shown PrEP can reduce the risk of acquiring HIV by more than 90% through sex or injection drug use (Anderson et al., 2012; Centers for Disease Control and Prevention, 2021). Recently, the FDA approved a long-acting injectable version of PrEP called Apretude that provides an alternative to daily oral PrEP by requiring injections only once every two months, reducing adherence challenges and offering a more convenient prevention option. Similarly, post-exposure prophylaxis (PEP) involves taking antiretroviral medicines within 72 hours after a potential HIV exposure to prevent infection. Recently, "Doxy-PEP," short for doxycycline post-exposure prophylaxis, involves the use of the antibiotic doxycycline after potential exposure via condomless sex to reduce the likelihood of acquiring chlamydia, syphilis, and/or gonorrhea (Bolan et al., 2015; Grant et al., 2020). Prevention scientists are cautiously optimistic about

Doxy-PEP's potential as part of a comprehensive STI prevention strategy as studies show promising results, particularly among high-risk populations. As the evidence grows, Doxy-PEP could become a valuable tool in reducing the burden of STIs (and therefore support HIV prevention) among Black SMM.

Research is also exploring other innovative preventive drug formulations and modalities, including implants that release medication over extended periods can provide a discreet and low-maintenance option for HIV prevention. Scientists are also developing, topical applications such as rectal microbicide gels that offer localized protection. The ongoing research and pilot programs are crucial for understanding the long-term efficacy and safety of this biomedical intervention. Other innovations such as longer-acting injectables and HIV/STI vaccines hold great promise for the future. These advancements can provide more options for individuals to protect themselves against disease. However, there are still concerns about the potential development of antibiotic resistance and side effects associated with long-term antibiotic use (Unemo et al., 2019). As research progresses, it will be crucial to integrate these new technologies into existing prevention science frameworks to maximize their impact on community health for Black SMM.

Treatment as Prevention

Treatment as prevention (also known as TasP) is a public health framework and strategy to reduce HIV incidence by treating individuals with ART to maintain an undetectable viral load to prevent transmission to others (CDC, 2023; National Institute of Allergy and Infectious Diseases, 2019). The basis for this approach relies on the knowledge that when HIV viral load is reduced to undetectable levels in the blood through consistent ART, the risk of transmitting the virus to sexual partners is effectively zero. This concept is encapsulated in the U=U campaign (Undetectable = Untransmittable), which has been pivotal in reducing the stigma associated with HIV (National Institute of Allergy and Infectious Diseases, 2019). By effectively reducing the viral load to undetectable levels, TasP not only improves the health outcomes of people living with HIV but also plays a crucial role in preventing the spread of the virus within the community.

Behavioral Interventions

Behavioral interventions address risk behaviors that contribute to HIV/STI transmission and acquisition. Comprehensive education and counseling are fundamental components of these interventions. For example, the "Many Men, Many Voices" (3MV) and "d-up: Defend Yourself!" programs are two evidence-based behavioral interventions aimed at preventing HIV among Black gay men. 3MV is a group-level intervention designed to address the unique cultural, social, and psychological factors influencing HIV risk in Black gay and bisexual men (Wilton et al., 2009). It involves a series of group sessions that cover a range of topics, including self-esteem, racial and sexual identity, HIV knowledge, and communication skills to increase condom use and HIV testing. "d-up: Defend Yourself!" is a community-level intervention that utilizes peer volunteers to lead community mobilization efforts and promote HIV prevention through cultural and social activities (Jones et al., 2008). This program focuses on increasing awareness and knowledge about HIV, promoting safer sex practices, and reducing stigma within the community. Peer volunteers are trained to become community advocates who organize events and create educational materials tailored to the cultural context of Black SMM. Both interventions leverage community engagement and peer support to foster sustainable behavior changes and improve health outcomes among Black SMM. These and other behavioral interventions can significantly reduce HIV/STI transmission rates and improve overall sexual health among Black gay and bisexual men through a combination of comprehensive education, personalized counseling, and community engagement. For example, the HIV Prevention Trials Network (HPTN) 073 provided Black SMM with PrEP alongside client-centered care coordination, which included personalized counseling and support (Nelson et al., 2022; Wheeler et al., 2019); findings showed that PrEP was well-accepted evidenced by 79% uptake within one month. This underscores the importance of integrating behavioral interventions with biomedical strategies like PrEP, as this combination can further enhance HIV prevention efforts and reduce the disparities experienced by Black gay and bisexual men.

Structural Interventions

Structural interventions address the broader social, economic, and environmental factors that influence HIV/STI risk. One type of structural intervention involves enacting policies and legislation that protect the rights of vulnerable populations and promote access to healthcare services (Adimora & Auerbach, 2010), such as, anti-discrimination laws and policies that ensure healthcare access regardless of sexual orientation or gender identity. Some approaches focus on improving the social determinants of health, such as housing stability and employment opportunities. Other structural interventions involve expansive billing practices and flexible hours of operation in healthcare organizations to improve access to care for marginalized or low-resourced individuals (Brown et al., 2019; Sipe et al., 2017). Integrating additional services such as mental health and substance use treatment within primary care settings is also a structural intervention that can address co-occurring conditions that exacerbate HIV/STI risks in communities. Ensuring equitable access to resources and services is key to optimal structural interventions (Bowleg et al., 2022; Fauci et al., 2019).

Technological Innovations

Advances in technology are increasingly shaping the future of HIV/STI prevention. For example, telemedicine has emerged as a powerful and acceptable tool to expand access to prevention and treatment services by offering remote consultations and follow-ups to mitigate some geographical and structural barriers and provide timely care to those in need. Other digital health tools such as mobile apps and online platforms have also proliferated and offer a significant contribution to prevention. These tools can offer education, risk assessments, social support, and linkages to services, enhancing the reach and effectiveness of HIV/STI prevention efforts. Telehealth platforms and mobile health (mHealth) applications have made it easier for Black SMM (along with the general population) to receive confidential medical consultations, obtain prescriptions for PrEP and HIV treatment, and access mental health support (Lee & Valerius, 2020; Muessig et al., 2017; Wong et al., 2020). Additionally, online communities and social media platforms have created spaces for Black SMM to share experiences, receive peer support, and engage in educational campaigns about sexual health and HIV prevention (Holloway et al., 2017). Mobile smartphone apps like "HealthMpowerment" provide tailored health resources and support networks, empowering users with the information needed to make informed health decisions (Hightow-Weidman et al., 2018). These technological advancements have collectively contributed to reducing health disparities and promoting better sexual health outcomes by increasing access to crucial health services and information. As technology continues to evolve, it holds the potential to transform HIV/STI prevention on a broader scale, making healthcare more accessible, personalized, and effective for those most at risk.

US Strategic Plans

Given the current HIV/STI prevention and treatment landscape, the USA launched the Ending the HIV Epidemic (EHE) plan for America in 2019 to address the ongoing public health challenges posed by HIV. The EHE aims to reduce new HIV infections by 90% by 2030 through four key strategies. These include diagnosing people with HIV as early as possible and treating those living with HIV quickly to achieve viral suppression. The plan also focuses on preventing new cases using PrEP and syringe services programs and responding swiftly to potential HIV outbreaks (Fauci et al., 2019; Office of Infectious Disease and HIV/AIDS Policy, HHS, 2020). Similarly, the National STI Strategic Plan was introduced in 2021 to address the increasing STI incidence by improving targeted research, addressing social determinants of STIs, and fostering a comprehensive, coordinated response to the STI epidemic across multiple sectors and stakeholders (U.S. Department of Health and Human Services, 2020). Both plans emphasize the importance of enhancing data collection and use, increasing public awareness and education, ensuring equitable access to healthcare services, and community engagement. These two agendas are important areas to consider since combined they create opportunities to consider more well-rounded approaches to sexual minority health. Moreover, the National HIV/AIDS Strategy for the USA has highlighted the sexual practices of SMM as a topic in need of additional high-quality research and the National Institutes of Health announced an exclusive strategy for preventing HIV infections by prioritizing access to and utilization of biomedical prevention tools (National Institutes of Health Office of AIDS Research, 2015, 2018). This integrated approach underscores the importance of culturally competent care and the need for ongoing community engagement to ensure that the benefits of these national strategies are equitably distributed, thereby fostering a more inclusive public health landscape. Collectively, these initiatives represent an intentional effort to mitigate HIV/STI disparities and improve health outcomes in a comprehensive way. Therefore, it is crucial to integrate these strategic frameworks into targeted prevention science for Black SMM. This approach will not only help reduce HIV/STI rates but also address the unique social, cultural, and structural challenges faced by Black SMM. Prevention science can make significant strides toward closing the gap in health disparities and ensuring that Black SMM receive the full benefits of these national efforts.

Overview of this Handbook

The significance of HIV/STI epidemiology and scientific advancement underscores the need for focused and culturally competent approaches to support the sexual health of Black SMM. However, innovative and consistent methods to engage and retain this community in research, clinical care, and prevention behaviors lag substantially. Medical mistrust remains prevalent and Black SMM consistently report feeling that researchers and clinicians do not care about them and misunderstand their needs (Cahill et al., 2017; Dangerfield II et al., 2022; Dangerfield II et al., 2021; Quinn et al., 2018). Additionally, new approaches through digital platforms post-COVID are eclipsing traditional research and community engagement methods and contemporary strategies to engage racial and sexual minority groups are not well understood. Therefore, this handbook draws on 10 years of significant research from Dangerfield II et al. involving Black SMM and provides advanced and contemporary methodology for sexual health prevention science for this key population. Chapter 1 focuses on the sexual epidemiology of Black gay and bisexual men, examining the prevalence and patterns of HIV and other STIs within this population. Chapter 2 redefines traditional risk concepts, theorizes sexual health behavior, and identifies critical research questions that need addressing to improve health outcomes. Chapter 3 discusses effective strategies for recruiting, retaining, and engaging Black SMM in STI/HIV prevention research, highlighting the importance of culturally sensitive approaches. Chapter 4 introduces person-centered statistical approaches for designing studies and interventions, offering innovative methods to tailor prevention efforts. Chapter 5 emphasizes the importance of contemporary and culturally responsive qualitative methodologies to capture the lived experiences of Black SMM. Chapter 6 explores the role of peer change agents as both behavioral and structural interventionists, underscoring their impact on health behavior change. Chapter 7 delves into targeted and tailored sexual health communication strategies, emphasizing the need for messages that resonate with Black SMM. Chapter 8 addresses the pervasive issue of sexual health misinformation and strategies to combat its spread. Chapter 9 outlines the ethical considerations necessary for conducting research with Black sexual minority men, ensuring that studies are both respectful and beneficial to the community. Finally, Chap. 10 proposes next steps for advancing sexual health prevention science and methodology, advocating for more inclusive and holistic research to support minority sexual health.

This handbook identifies knowledge gaps and proposes ideas and recommendations for innovative methods and perspectives to enhance the reach of existing and novel prevention tools for this community. Researchers, clinicians, and disease prevention practitioners will be guided through sexual health research and intervention design processes using novel and successful studies among Black SMM to design effective, evidence-based, and ethical strategies that address unique challenges, improve health outcomes, and reduce disparities in HIV/STI prevention and treatment within this marginalized population. This handbook serves as a resource for training and developing both emerging and experienced prevention scientists and clinicians. It offers innovative ideas to help current experts refine and improve intervention methods for disease prevention in the USA and globally. In addition to offering practical tools and strategies, this handbook also serves as a resource for fostering a deeper understanding of the sociocultural dynamics that influence health behaviors and outcomes among Black SMM. By bridging theoretical knowledge with real-world applications, this handbook aims to empower prevention scientists and public health professionals to create more inclusive and effective health interventions that are responsive to the evolving needs of this community. The theoretical and methodological approaches presented in this text can also be used as a guide for targeted approaches for other vulnerable subgroups, broadening its applicability. Ultimately, it seeks to contribute to a more holistic prevention science framework where Black SMM are provided the highest standards of research, engagement, and care.

References

Adimora, A. A., & Auerbach, J. D. (2010). Structural interventions for HIV prevention in the United States. *JAIDS Journal of Acquired Immune Deficiency Syndromes*, *55*, S132–S135. https://doi.org/10.1097/QAI.0b013e3181fbcb38

Anderson, P. L., Glidden, D. V., Liu, A., Buchbinder, S., Lama, J. R., Guanira, J. V., McMahan, V., Bushman, L. R., Casapía, M., Montoya-Herrera, O., Veloso, V. G., Mayer, K. H., Chariyalertsak, S., Schechter, M., Bekker, L.-G., Kallás, E. G., Grant, R. M., & Team, F. the iPrEx S. (2012). Emtricitabine-tenofovir concentrations and pre-exposure prophylaxis efficacy in men who have sex with men. *Science Translational Medicine*, *4*(151), 151ra125–151ra125. https://doi.org/10.1126/scitranslmed.3004006

Bernstein, K. T., Marcus, J. L., Nieri, G., Philip, S. S., & Klausner, J. D. (2010). Rectal gonorrhea and chlamydia reinfection is associated with increased risk of HIV seroconversion: *JAIDS Journal of Acquired Immune Deficiency Syndromes*, *53*(4), 537–543. https://doi.org/10.1097/QAI.0b013e3181c3ef29

Bolan, R. K., Beymer, M. R., Weiss, R. E., Flynn, R. P., Leibowitz, A. A., & Klausner, J. D. (2015). Doxycycline prophylaxis to reduce incident syphilis among HIV-infected men who have sex with men who continue to engage in high risk sex: A randomized, controlled pilot study. *Sexually Transmitted Diseases*, *42*(2), 98–103. https://doi.org/10.1097/OLQ.0000000000000216

Bond, J. C., & Ford, J. V. (2024). A call for sex-positive epidemiology. *American Journal of Epidemiology*, kwae054. https://doi.org/10.1093/aje/kwae054

Bonett, S., Dowshen, N., Bauermeister, J., Meanley, S., Wirtz, A. L., Celentano, D. D., Galai, N., Arrington-Sanders, R., & the PUSH Study Group. (2021). Characterizing the PrEP continuum for Black and Latinx sexual and gender Minority Youth. *AIDS and Behavior 26,* 1211–1221. https://doi.org/10.1007/s10461-021-03476-6

Bowleg, L., Malekzadeh, A. N., Mbaba, M., & Boone, C. A. (2022). Ending the HIV epidemic for all, not just some: Structural racism as a fundamental but overlooked social-structural determinant of the US HIV epidemic. *Current Opinion in HIV and AIDS*, *17*(2), 40–45. https://doi.org/10.1097/COH.0000000000000724

Brown, A. F., Ma, G. X., Miranda, J., Eng, E., Castille, D., Brockie, T., Jones, P., Airhihenbuwa, C. O., Farhat, T., Zhu, L., & Trinh-Shevrin, C. (2019). Structural interventions to reduce and eliminate health disparities. *American Journal of Public Health*, *109*(S1), S72–S78. https://doi.org/10.2105/AJPH.2018.304844

Burns, P. A., Mena, L. A., & Crosby, R. L. (2020). Foretelling the future: Predicting STI diagnosis and its implications for Ending the HIV epidemic among Black men who have sex with men. *Journal of Urban Health*. https://doi.org/10.1007/s11524-019-00413-w

Cahill, S., Taylor, S. W., Elsesser, S. A., Mena, L., Hickson, D., & Mayer, K. H. (2017). Stigma, medical mistrust, and perceived racism may affect PrEP awareness and uptake in black compared to white gay and bisexual men in Jackson, Mississippi and Boston, Massachusetts. *AIDS Care*, *29*(11), 1351–1358. https://doi.org/10.1080/09540121.2017.1300633

Centers for Disease Control and Prevention. (2016, January 1). *Reported STDs Reach All-time High for 6th Consecutive Year*. CDC. https://www.cdc.gov/media/releases/2021/p0413-stds.html

Centers for Disease Control and Prevention. (2017). *Sexually Transmitted Disease Surveillance 2016*. https://www.cdc.gov/std/stats16/CDC_2016_STDS_Report-for508WebSep21_2017_1644.pdf

Centers for Disease Control and Prevention. (2020, February 4). *HIV and African American Gay and Bisexual Men | HIV by Group | HIV/AIDS | CDC*. https://www.cdc.gov/hiv/group/msm/bmsm.html

Centers for Disease Control and Prevention. (2021, May 13). *PrEP Effectiveness | PrEP | HIV Basics | HIV/AIDS | CDC*. https://www.cdc.gov/hiv/basics/prep/prep-effectiveness.html

Centers for Disease Control and Prevention. (2023, August 9). *HIV Treatment as Prevention | HIV Risk and Prevention | HIV/AIDS | CDC*. https://www.cdc.gov/hiv/risk/art/index.html

Chesson, H. W., Song, R., Bingham, A., & Farnham, P. G. (2021). The estimated number and lifetime medical cost of HIV infections attributable to sexually transmitted infections acquired in the United States in 2018: A compilation of published modeling results. *Sexually Transmitted Diseases*, *48*(4), 292. https://doi.org/10.1097/OLQ.0000000000001358

Coleman, J. D., Tate, A. D., Gaddist, B., & White, J. (2016). Social determinants of HIV-related stigma in faith-based organizations. *American Journal of Public Health*, *106*(3), 492–496. https://doi.org/10.2105/AJPH.2015.302985

Craib, K. J., Meddings, D. R., Strathdee, S. A., Hogg, R. S., Montaner, J. S., O'Shaughnessy, M. V., & Schechter, M. T. (1995). Rectal gonorrhoea as an independent risk factor for HIV infection in a cohort of homosexual men. *Genitourinary Medicine*, *71*(3), 150–154. https://doi.org/10.1136/sti.71.3.150

Dangerfield II, D. T., Anderson, J. N., Wylie, C., Arrington-Sanders, R., Bluthenthal, R. N., Beyrer, C., & Farley, J. E. (2022). Refining a multicomponent intervention to increase perceived HIV risk and PrEP initiation: Focus group study among Black sexual minority men. *JMIR Formative Research*, *6*(8), e34181. https://doi.org/10.2196/34181

Dangerfield II, D. T., Cooper, J., Heidari, O., Allen, S., Winder, T. J. A., & Lucas, G. M. (2021). Nursing and health care preferences among opioid and stimulant using Black sexual minority men: An exploratory study. *Journal of the Association of Nurses in AIDS Care*, *32*(5), e30–e39. https://doi.org/10.1097/JNC.0000000000000201

Dean, H. D., & Fenton, K. A. (2010). Addressing social determinants of health in the prevention and control of HIV/AIDS, viral Hepatitis, sexually transmitted infections, and tuberculosis. *Public Health Reports*, *125*(Suppl 4), 1–5.

Deguchi, T., Yasuda, M., & Ito, S. (2012). Management of pharyngeal gonorrhea is crucial to prevent the emergence and spread of antibiotic-resistant Neisseria gonorrhoeae. *Antimicrobial Agents and Chemotherapy*, *56*(7), 4039–4040. https://doi.org/10.1128/AAC.00505-12

Eisinger, R. W., Dieffenbach, C. W., & Fauci, A. S. (2019). HIV viral load and transmissibility of HIV infection: Undetectable equals Untransmittable. *JAMA*, *321*(5), 451–452. https://doi.org/10.1001/jama.2018.21167

Etheridge, T., Bowen, R. C., Raven, M., Snow, K. B., Urban, A. W., & Chang, J. S. (2019). *Ocular Syphilis: Clinical Manifestations and Treatment Course, 118*(4), 6.

Fauci, A. S., Redfield, R. R., Sigounas, G., Weahkee, M. D., & Giroir, B. P. (2019). Ending the HIV Epidemic: A Plan for the United States. *JAMA*, *321*(9), 844. https://doi.org/10.1001/jama.2019.1343

Fishbein, M., & Yzer, M. C. (2003). Using theory to design effective health behavior interventions. *Communication Theory*, *13*(2), 164–183. https://doi.org/10.1111/j.1468-2885.2003.tb00287.x

Fleming, D. T., & Wasserheit, J. N. (1999). From epidemiological synergy to public health policy and practice: The contribution of other sexually transmitted diseases to sexual transmission of HIV infection. *Sexually Transmitted Infections*, *75*(1), 3–17.

Gaspari, V., Marangoni, A., D'Antuono, A., Roncarati, G., Salvo, M., Foschi, C., & Re, M. C. (2019). Pharyngeal chlamydia and gonorrhea: A hidden problem. *International Journal of STD & AIDS*, 095646241983892. https://doi.org/10.1177/0956462419838922

Grant, J. S., Stafylis, C., Celum, C., Grennan, T., Haire, B., Kaldor, J., Luetkemeyer, A. F., Saunders, J. M., Molina, J.-M., & Klausner, J. D. (2020). Doxycycline prophylaxis for bacterial sexually transmitted infections. *Clinical Infectious Diseases*, *70*(6), 1247–1253. https://doi.org/10.1093/cid/ciz866

Hess, K. L., Hu, X., Lansky, A., Mermin, J., & Hall, H. I. (2017). Lifetime risk of a diagnosis of HIV infection in the United States. *Annals of Epidemiology*, *27*(4), 238–243. https://doi.org/10.1016/j.annepidem.2017.02.003

Hightow-Weidman, L., Muessig, K., Knudtson, K., Srivatsa, M., Lawrence, E., LeGrand, S., Hotten, A., & Hosek, S. (2018). A gamified smartphone app to support engagement in care and medication adherence for HIV-positive young men who have sex with men (AllyQuest): Development and pilot study. *JMIR Public Health and Surveillance*, *4*(2), e34. https://doi.org/10.2196/publichealth.8923

Holloway, I. W., Winder, T. J., Lea III, C. H., Tan, D., Boyd, D., & Novak, D. (2017). Technology use and preferences for mobile phone–based HIV prevention and treatment among Black young men who have sex with men: Exploratory research. *JMIR mHealth and uHealth*, *5*(4), e46. https://doi.org/10.2196/mhealth.6436

Hoots, B. E., Finlayson, T. J., Wejnert, C., Paz-Bailey, G., & National HIV Behavioral Surveillance (NHBS) Study Group. (2017). Updated data on linkage to human immunodeficiency virus care and antiretroviral treatment among men who have sex with men-20 Cities, United States. *The Journal of Infectious Diseases*, *216*(7), 808–812. https://doi.org/10.1093/infdis/jix007

Jeffries IV, W. L., Dailey, A., Jin, C., Carter, J., & Scales, L. (2020). Trends in diagnosis of HIV infection, linkage to medical care, and viral suppression among men who have sex with men, by race/ethnicity and age—33 Jurisdictions, United States, 2014–2018. *MMWR. Morbidity and Mortality Weekly Report*, *69*. https://doi.org/10.15585/mmwr.mm6938a1

Johnson Jones, M., Chapin-Bardales, J., Bizune, D., et al. (2019). Extragenital chlamydia and gonorrhea among community venue–attending men who have sex with men—Five Cities, United States, 2017 | MMWR. *MMWR Morb Mortal Wkly Rep*, *68*, 321–325.

Jones, K. T., Gray, P., Whiteside, Y. O., Wang, T., Bost, D., Dunbar, E., Foust, E., & Johnson, W. D. (2008). Evaluation of an HIV prevention intervention adapted for Black men who have sex with men. *American Journal of Public Health*, *98*(6), 1043–1050. https://doi.org/10.2105/AJPH.2007.120337

Koblin, B. A., Mayer, K. H., Eshleman, S. H., Wang, L., Mannheimer, S., del Rio, C., Shoptaw, S., Magnus, M., Buchbinder, S., Wilton, L., Liu, T.-Y., Cummings, V., Piwowar-Manning, E., Fields, S. D., Griffith, S., Elharrar, V., & Wheeler, D. (2013). Correlates of HIV acquisition in a cohort of Black men who have sex with men in the United States: HIV Prevention Trials Network (HPTN) 061. *PLoS ONE*, *8*(7), e70413. https://doi.org/10.1371/journal.pone.0070413

Lee, S. B., & Valerius, J. (2020). mHealth interventions to promote anti-retroviral adherence in HIV: Narrative review. *JMIR mHealth and uHealth*, *8*(8), e14739. https://doi.org/10.2196/14739

Li, X., Li, M., Yang, Y., Zhong, X., Feng, B., Xin, H., Li, Z., Jin, Q., & Gao, L. (2016). Anal HPV/HIV co-infection among Men Who Have Sex with Men: A cross-sectional survey from three cities in China. *Scientific Reports*, *6*, 21368. https://doi.org/10.1038/srep21368

Lin, C., Franceschi, S., & Clifford, G. M. (2017). Human papillomavirus types from infection to cancer in the anus, according to sex and HIV status: A systematic review and meta-analysis. *The Lancet Infectious Diseases*. https://doi.org/10.1016/S1473-3099(17)30653-9

Machalek, D. A., Tao, Y., Shilling, H., Jensen, J. S., Unemo, M., Murray, G., Chow, E. P. F., Low, N., Garland, S. M., Vodstrcil, L. A., Fairley, C. K., Hocking, J. S., Zhang, L., & Bradshaw, C. S. (2020). Prevalence of mutations associated with resistance to macrolides and fluoroquinolones in Mycoplasma genitalium: A systematic review and meta-analysis. *The Lancet Infectious Diseases*, *20*(11), 1302–1314. https://doi.org/10.1016/S1473-3099(20)30154-7

Maulsby, C., Millett, G., Lindsey, K., Kelley, R., Johnson, K., Montoya, D., & Holtgrave, D. (2013). A systematic review of HIV interventions for Black men who have sex with men (MSM). *BMC Public Health*, *13*, 625. https://doi.org/10.1186/1471-2458-13-625

Mayer, K. H., & Venkatesh, K. K. (2011). Interactions of HIV, other sexually transmitted diseases, and genital tract inflammation facilitating local pathogen transmission and acquisition. *American Journal of Reproductive Immunology (New York, N.Y. : 1989)*, *65*(3), 308–316. https://doi.org/10.1111/j.1600-0897.2010.00942.x

Millett, G. A., Peterson, J. L., Flores, S. A., Hart, T. A., Jeffries 4th, W. L., Wilson, P. A., Rourke, S. B., Heilig, C. M., Elford, J., Fenton, K. A., & Remis, R. S. (2012). Comparisons of disparities and risks of HIV infection in black and other men who have sex with men in Canada, UK, and USA: A meta-analysis. *The Lancet*, *380*(9839), 341–348. https://doi.org/10.1016/S0140-6736(12)60899-X

Millett, G. A., Peterson, J. L., Wolitski, R. J., & Stall, R. (2006). Greater risk for HIV infection of Black men who have sex with men: A critical literature review. *American Journal of Public Health*, *96*(6), 1007–1019. https://doi.org/10.2105/AJPH.2005.066720

Muessig, K. E., LeGrand, S., Horvath, K. J., Bauermeister, J. A., & Hightow-Weidman, L. B. (2017). Recent mHealth interventions to support medication adherence among HIV-positive men who have sex with men. *Current Opinion in HIV and AIDS*, *12*(5), 432–441. https://doi.org/10.1097/COH.0000000000000401

Mustanski, B., Feinstein, B. A., Madkins, K., Sullivan, P. D., & Swann, G. (2017). Prevalence and risk factors for rectal and urethral sexually transmitted infections from self-collected samples among young men who have sex with men participating in the Keep It Up! 2.0 randomized controlled trial. *Sexually Transmitted Diseases*, *44*(8), 483–488. https://doi.org/10.1097/OLQ.0000000000000636

National Institues of Health Office of AIDS Research. (2015, August 12). *NOT-OD-15-137: NIH HIV/AIDS Research Priorities and Guidelines for Determining AIDS Funding*. http://grants.nih.gov/grants/guide/notice-files/NOT-OD-15-137.html
National Institues of Health Office of AIDS Research. (2018). *Trans-NIH Strategic Plan for HIV and HIV-Related Research*. 13.
National Institute of Allergy and Infectious Diseases. (2019, May 21). *HIV Undetectable=Untransmittable (U=U), or Treatment as Prevention*. https://www.niaid.nih.gov/diseases-conditions/treatment-prevention
Nelson, L. E., Wilton, L., Whitfield, D. L., Williams, G. C., Mayer, K. H., Komárek, A., Boyd, D. T., Beauchamp, G., Fields, S. D., Wheeler, D. P., & for the HPTN 073 Study Team. (2022). Client-Centered Care Coordination (C4™) for HIV/STI Prevention: A theoretical, conceptual, and methodological overview—HIV Prevention Trials Network (HPTN) 073. *Sexuality Research and Social Policy*. https://doi.org/10.1007/s13178-022-00687-x
Office of Infectious Disease and HIV/AIDS Policy, HHS. (2020, February). *Ending the HIV Epidemic: A Plan for America*. https://www.hiv.gov/federal-response/ending-the-hiv-epidemic/overview#:~:text=Ending%20the%20HIV%20Epidemic%3A%20A%20Plan%20for%20America%20(EHE),United%20States%20within%2010%20years
Office of the Surgeon General (US) & Office of Population Affairs (US). (2001). *The Surgeon General's Call to Action to Promote Sexual Health and Responsible Sexual Behavior*. Office of the Surgeon General (US). http://www.ncbi.nlm.nih.gov/books/NBK44216/
Patton, M. E., Kidd, S., Llata, E., Stenger, M., Braxton, J., Asbel, L., Bernstein, K., Gratzer, B., Jespersen, M., Kerani, R., Mettenbrink, C., Mohamed, M., Pathela, P., Schumacher, C., Stirland, A., Stover, J., Tabidze, I., Kirkcaldy, R. D., & Weinstock, H. (2014). Extragenital gonorrhea and chlamydia testing and infection among men who have sex with men—STD Surveillance Network, United States, 2010–2012. *Clinical Infectious Diseases*, *58*(11), 1564–1570. https://doi.org/10.1093/cid/ciu184
Piketty, C., Selinger-Leneman, H., Grabar, S., Duvivier, C., Bonmarchand, M., Abramowitz, L., Costagliola, D., & Mary-Krause, M. (2008). Marked increase in the incidence of invasive anal cancer among HIV-infected patients despite treatment with combination antiretroviral therapy. *AIDS*, *22*(10), 1203–1211. https://doi.org/10.1097/QAD.0b013e3283023f78
Pitasi, M. A. (2021). Vital signs: HIV infection, diagnosis, treatment, and prevention among gay, bisexual, and other men who have sex with men – United States, 2010–2019. *MMWR. Morbidity and Mortality Weekly Report*, *70*. https://doi.org/10.15585/mmwr.mm7048e1
Poteat, T. C., & Logie, C. H. (2022). A case for strengths-based approaches to addressing intersectional stigma in HIV research. *American Journal of Public Health*, *112*(S4), S347–S349. https://doi.org/10.2105/AJPH.2021.306659
Quinn, K., Dickson-Gomez, J., Zarwell, M., Pearson, B., & Lewis, M. (2018). "A gay man and a doctor are just like, a recipe for destruction": How racism and homonegativity in healthcare settings influence PrEP uptake among young Black MSM. *AIDS and Behavior, 23,* 1951–1963. https://doi.org/10.1007/s10461-018-2375-z
Rosenstock, I. M. (1974). Historical Origins of the Health Belief Model. *Health Education Monographs*, *2*(4), 328–335. https://doi.org/10.1177/109019817400200403
Rottingen, J.-A., William, C., & Garnett, G. (2001). A systematic review of the epidemiologic interactions between class sexually transmitted diseases and HIV: How much Is really known? *Sexually Transmitted Diseases*, *28*(10), 579–597.
Schackman, B. R., Fleishman, J. A., Su, A. E., Berkowitz, B. K., Moore, R. D., Walensky, R. P., Becker, J. E., Voss, C., Paltiel, A. D., Weinstein, M. C., Freedberg, K. A., Gebo, K. A., & Losina, E. (2015). The lifetime medical cost savings from preventing HIV in the United States. *Medical Care*, *53*(4), 293–301. https://doi.org/10.1097/MLR.0000000000000308
Scott-Sheldon, L. A. J., & Chan, P. A. (2020). Increasing sexually transmitted infections in the U.S.: A call for action for research, clinical, and public health practice. *Archives of Sexual Behavior*, *49*(1), 13–17. https://doi.org/10.1007/s10508-019-01584-y

Sharpe, T. T., Voûte, C., Rose, M. A., Cleveland, J., Dean, H. D., & Fenton, K. (2011). Social determinants of HIV/AIDS and sexually transmitted diseases among Black women: Implications for health equity. *Journal of Women's Health*, *21*(3), 249–254. https://doi.org/10.1089/jwh.2011.3350

Shover, C. L., Javanbakht, M., Shoptaw, S., Bolan, R. K., Lee, S.-J., Parsons, J. T., Rendina, J., & Gorbach, P. M. (2018). HIV preexposure prophylaxis initiation at a large community clinic: Differences between eligibility, awareness, and uptake. *American Journal of Public Health*, *108*(10), 1408–1417. https://doi.org/10.2105/AJPH.2018.304623

Sipe, T. A., Barham, T. L., Johnson, W. D., Joseph, H. A., Tungol-Ashmon, M. L., & O'Leary, A. (2017). Structural interventions in HIV prevention: A taxonomy and descriptive systematic review. *AIDS and Behavior*, *21*(12), 3366–3430. https://doi.org/10.1007/s10461-017-1965-5

Solomon, M. M., Mayer, K. H., Glidden, D. V., Liu, A. Y., McMahan, V. M., Guanira, J. V., Chariyalertsak, S., Fernandez, T., Grant, R. M., Bekker, L.-G., Buchbinder, S., Casapia, M., Chariyalertsak, S., Guanira, J., Kallas, E., Lama, J., Mayer, K., Montoya, O., Schechter, M., & Veloso, V. (2014). Syphilis predicts HIV incidence among men and transgender women who have sex with men in a preexposure prophylaxis trial. *Clinical Infectious Diseases*, *59*(7), 1020–1026. https://doi.org/10.1093/cid/ciu450

Sullivan, P. S., Knox, J., Jones, J., Taussig, J., Graves, M. V., Millett, G., Luisi, N., Hall, E., Sanchez, T. H., Rio, C. D., Kelley, C., Rosenberg, E. S., & Guest, J. L. (2021). Understanding disparities in viral suppression among Black MSM living with HIV in Atlanta Georgia. *Journal of the International AIDS Society*, *24*(4), e25689. https://doi.org/10.1002/jia2.25689

Sullivan, P. S., Rosenberg, E. S., Sanchez, T. H., Kelley, C. F., Luisi, N., Cooper, H. L., Diclemente, R. J., Wingood, G. M., Frew, P. M., Salazar, L. F., Del Rio, C., Mulligan, M. J., & Peterson, J. L. (2015). Explaining racial disparities in HIV incidence in black and white men who have sex with men in Atlanta, GA: A prospective observational cohort study. *Annals of Epidemiology*, *25*(6), 445–454. https://doi.org/10.1016/j.annepidem.2015.03.006

Unemo, M., Golparian, D., & Eyre, D. W. (2019). Antimicrobial resistance in Neisseria gonorrhoeae and treatment of gonorrhea. In M. Christodoulides (Ed.), *Neisseria gonorrhoeae: Methods and Protocols* (pp. 37–58). Springer. https://doi.org/10.1007/978-1-4939-9496-0_3

Unemo, M., & Jensen, J. S. (2017). Antimicrobial-resistant sexually transmitted infections: Gonorrhoea and Mycoplasma genitalium. *Nature Reviews Urology*, *14*(3), Article 3. https://doi.org/10.1038/nrurol.2016.268

U.S. Department of Health and Human Services. (2020). *STI National Strategic Plan for the United States 2021-2025*. https://www.hhs.gov/sites/default/files/STI-National-Strategic-Plan-2021-2025.pdf

Volk, J. E., Marcus, J. L., Phengrasamy, T., Blechinger, D., Nguyen, D. P., Follansbee, S., & Hare, C. B. (2015). No new HIV infections with increasing use of HIV preexposure prophylaxis in a clinical practice setting. *Clinical Infectious Diseases*, *61*(10), 1601–1603. https://doi.org/10.1093/cid/civ778

Wasserheit, J. (1992). Epidemiological Synergy: Interrelationships between human immunodeficiency virus infection and other sexually transmitted diseases. *LWW*, *19*(2), 61–77.

Watson, R. J., Collibee, C., Maksut, J. L., Earnshaw, V. A., Rucinski, K., & Eaton, L. (2022). High levels of undiagnosed rectal STIs suggest that screening remains inadequate among Black gay, bisexual and other men who have sex with men. *Sexually Transmitted Infections*, *98*(2), 125–127. https://doi.org/10.1136/sextrans-2020-054563

Wheeler, D. P., Fields, S. D., Beauchamp, G., Chen, Y. Q., Emel, L. M., Hightow-Weidman, L., Hucks-Ortiz, C., Kuo, I., Lucas, J., Magnus, M., Mayer, K. H., Nelson, L. E., Hendrix, C. W., Piwowar-Manning, E., Shoptaw, S., Watkins, P., Watson, C. C., & Wilton, L. (2019). Pre-exposure prophylaxis initiation and adherence among Black men who have sex with men (MSM) in three US cities: Results from the HPTN 073 study. *Journal of the International AIDS Society*, *22*(2), e25223. https://doi.org/10.1002/jia2.25223

Wilton, L., Herbst, J. H., Coury-Doniger, P., Painter, T. M., English, G., Alvarez, M. E., Scahill, M., Roberson, M. A., Lucas, B., Johnson, W. D., & Carey, J. W. (2009). Efficacy of an HIV/STI prevention intervention for Black men who have sex with men: Findings from the Many Men, Many Voices (3MV) Project. *AIDS and Behavior, 13*(3), 532–544. https://doi.org/10.1007/s10461-009-9529-y

Wong, K. Y. K., Stafylis, C., & Klausner, J. D. (2020). Telemedicine: A solution to disparities in human immunodeficiency virus prevention and pre-exposure prophylaxis uptake, and a framework to scalability and equity. *mHealth, 6*. https://doi.org/10.21037/mhealth.2019.12.06

Wood, B. R., & Guthrie, B. L. (2022). Recurrent bacterial sexually transmitted infections: Lessons from an HIV preexposure prophylaxis trial. *AIDS, 36*(8), 1191. https://doi.org/10.1097/QAD.0000000000003210

Workowski, K. A. (2021). Sexually Transmitted Infections Treatment Guidelines, 2021. *MMWR. Recommendations and Reports, 70*. https://doi.org/10.15585/mmwr.rr7004a1

World Health Organization. (2006). *Defining sexual health Report of a technical consultation on sexual health 28–31 January 2002, Geneva*. World Health Organization Press. https://www.cesas.lu/perch/resources/whodefiningsexualhealth.pdf

World Health Organization. (2024). *Sexual health*. https://www.who.int/health-topics/sexual-health

Zeggagh, J., Bauer, R., Delaugerre, C., Carette, D., Fressard, L., Charreau, I., Chidiac, C., Pialoux, G., Tremblay, C., Cua, E., Robineau, O., Raffi, F., Capitant, C., Spire, B., Meyer, L., & Molina, J. M. (2022). Incidence and risk factors for recurrent sexually transmitted infections among MSM on HIV pre-exposure prophylaxis. *AIDS, 36*(8), 1129–1134. https://doi.org/10.1097/QAD.0000000000003187

Contents

Chapter 1
The Sexual Epidemiology of Black Sexual Minority Men

Chapter Objectives

1. Conceptualize the discipline of sexual epidemiology within the prevention science landscape
2. Identify the significance of sexual epidemiology for HIV/STI prevention
3. Describe the sexual epidemiology of Black SMM and related significance in prevention science

Introduction to Sexual Epidemiology

Sexual health prevention science increased focus on improving sexual well-being within overall health (Anderson, 2013; Bond & Ford, 2024; Lefkowitz & Vasilenko, 2014). However, methodological approaches to study behavioral, psychological, social, and cultural dynamics among sexual minority men (SMM) are limited. Behavioral epidemiology studies the interplay between behaviors and health outcomes and provides a valuable lens to understand the patterns and determinants of sexual behaviors. However, there is a notable gap in the discipline regarding the sexual behaviors leading to disease and negative health outcomes, especially among Black gay, bisexual, and other Black SMM. Persistent health disparities suggest that scientists and public health practitioners need additional frameworks to better understand the precursors, activities, and changes in sexual behaviors and risk, especially for Black SMM. Applying the strengths of behavioral epidemiology to study sexual behaviors can further advance the prevention science and public health. Therefore, a novel and significant focus on "sexual epidemiology" is required.

Sexual epidemiology is a branch of behavioral epidemiology that examines the distribution, patterns, correlates, and determinants of sexual behavior within

D. T. Dangerfield II, *Prevention Science & Targeted Methods for HIV/STI Research with Black Sexual Minority Men*,
https://doi.org/10.1007/978-3-031-85130-8_1

populations (Dangerfield II, 2024). It investigates the precursors of sexual behaviors to understand diverse behaviors, experiences, and cultural dynamics that shape sexual practices and influence vulnerability within communities. Sexual epidemiology enhances prevention science by offering a focused approach to understanding how, why, and who engages in specific sexual behaviors. This field is crucial for prevention science because it provides needed insights into the patterns, determinants, and consequences of population health behavior. Results from this field can help researchers design targeted interventions to reduce negative health outcomes while promoting sexual well-being. Moreover, sexual epidemiology studies can improve comprehensive sexual education that covers topics that are relevant especially for marginalized minority groups and improve healthcare service models. Prevention scientists have emphasized the importance of comprehensive sexual health education, improved access to healthcare services, and integrating behavioral and biomedical approaches to prevent and manage STIs for more than a decade (Beyrer et al., 2012; Bond & Ford, 2024; Elopre et al., 2021; Sullivan et al., 2017). Incorporating sexual epidemiology into clinical training programs could improve clinical service delivery and targeted interventions. This comprehensive approach will help ensure that prevention efforts are equitable and inclusive, ultimately leading to healthier outcomes for everyone. As the field evolves, sexual epidemiology holds promise to inform research, intervention, and policy changes that prioritize key aspects of behavior for health equity.

Sexual Epidemiology Among Sexual Minority Men

Understanding the sexual practices and preferences among SMM is crucial for addressing public health disparities and designing culturally relevant interventions. A key area of focus in the sexual epidemiology of men who have sex with men involves sexual positioning practices. Sexual positioning practices include insertive anal intercourse (IAI), receptive anal intercourse (RAI), and oral sex (Dangerfield II et al., 2017b). Culturally, these behaviors are referred to as "top" (i.e., IAI) and "bottom" (i.e., RAI). Sexual positioning refers to the physical sexual practices (e.g., IAI, RAI, oral sex), while sexual roles refer to self-identified preferences or identities such as "top," "bottom," or "versatile" among SMM (Dangerfield II et al., 2017b). Additional terms such as "versatile bottom" and "versatile top" have also emerged among SMM (Dangerfield II et al., 2017a, 2018b; Truong et al., 2016). Culturally speaking, a "versatile bottom" primarily prefers RAI but occasionally practices IAI, while a "versatile top" mainly prefers IAI but sometimes participates in RAI depending upon the context (Truong et al., 2016). Sexual roles and related positioning practices play a significant part in shaping relationship dynamics and health behaviors among SMM generally but under-explored. Although it is essential to avoid reducing sexuality solely to disease outcomes, examining these behaviors within a public health framework is crucial for addressing the complex interplay between individual practices, social contexts, and cultural norms that influence well-being.

Focus on Black SMM

Prevention research generally falls short in representing Black SMM adequately. Many studies either have small sample sizes of Black SMM, include mixed race minority samples without considering cultural differences, or ignore role of race on sexuality in statistical models. Consequently, the literature lacks comprehensive insights regarding culture, sexuality, and health for Black SMM. An intentional focus on sexual epidemiology among Black SMM is crucial because of their unique and compounded social challenges relative to other U.S. populations including racism, discrimination, stigma, childhood adversity, socioeconomic challenges (Centers for Disease Control and Prevention (CDC), 2020). My research has specifically targeted sexual epidemiology for HIV and STI prevention for Black SMM (Dangerfield II et al., 2018b, 2018c, 2017a). These studies, among others, reveal the complex interplay between sexual behaviors, disease risk, and health. Understanding the specific behavioral, psychological, social, and cultural factors that influence sexuality and related health outcomes could help explain disparities and guide solutions.

Conceptual Framework for Sexual Epidemiology Among Black SM

According to the Theory of Gender and Power (Connell, 2014; Wingood & DiClemente, 2000) power dynamics based upon gender roles can create imbalances in decision-making ability regarding sexual practices and condom use in heterosexual partnerships. These expectations are complicated by a same-sex dynamic in which both partners are considered "men." The intersection of race, gender, and sexual orientation coupled with important psychological and social factors could result in unique experiences of marginalization for Black SMM, which can influence how they perceive and engage in sex. Additionally, societal pressures related to masculinity and gender norms can create internal conflicts around sexual identity, leading to complex sexual relationship dynamics that are not always easily understood or articulated. Because of this, some people might adopt sexual roles and practices that misalign with authentic preferences. Simon and Gagnon's (Simon & Gagnon, 1984) theory of sexual scripting suggests that sexual interactions can be informed by sexual "scripts" derived from cultural scenarios, interpersonal interactions, and intrapersonal characteristics that frame how people experience different sexual interactions. These scripts are further complicated by societal stigma, cultural expectations, and internalized homophobia, which can profoundly shape how Black SMM experience and express their sexual identities and behaviors.

To help advance and focus the field, we conducted a narrative review of the literature on sexual positioning practices among SMM and proposed a conceptual model examining the factors that influence power dynamics and sexual positioning in same-sex relationships (Dangerfield II et al., 2017b). The review suggested that broad psychological and social factors such as masculinity stereotypes, age, race/ethnicity, partner type, and HIV status influence sexual positioning preferences and the ability to mitigate risk. We adapted the model to better reflect cultural nuances among Black SMM (Dangerfield II et al., 2018c). Consistent with the original model, data suggested that personal preferences, partner type, and substance use influence sexual positioning among Black SMM. Additional psychological factors such as feelings of compromise, obligation, partner attraction, and HIV avoidance also emerged as key influences on sexual behaviors. We did not find that seeking masculine partners or using versatility was a means of regaining power in same-sex relationships as some might expect. Dynamics within the same-sex sexual encounter might not be power referring to physical or verbal ability, but could refer to power regarding personal agency regarding maintaining sexual preferences. Although some people might maintain their sexual positioning preferences, mutable factors such as partner type and substance use also shape sexual behavior and risk. Ultimately, identification with roles like "top," "bottom," or "versatile" does not fully predict behaviors or risk necessarily. Instead, unconscious motivations and assumptions within sexual relationships play a key understudied role in influencing behavior. Figure 1.1 shows a model hypothesizing how psychological, social, and contextual factors identified from previous frameworks affect sexual dynamics among Black SMM (Dangerfield II et al., 2017b, 2018c). These factors, which expanded the original models, highlight the complexity of sexual decision-making among Black SMM. Despite significant advances in understanding the sexual health behaviors of SMM, consistent measures to study sexual positioning, sexual roles, and the impact of sexual epidemiology on disease vulnerability still lag. There is also limited knowledge regarding the direction of the relationships among variables influencing sexual positioning and their implications for broader health outcomes other than HIV.

The Distribution of Sexual Positioning Practices Among Black SMM

Collectively, the literature shows range in self-reported roles and behaviors among Black SMM. Targeted studies show that **2%–25%** identify as 'bottom,' **0%–15%** as 'versatile bottom,' **4%–44%** as 'versatile,' **8%–10%** as 'versatile top,' and **8%–62%** identify as 'top' (Dangerfield II et al., 2017a, 2020; Wei & Raymond, 2010; Wilson et al., 2009). It is crucial to note that the literature on sexual roles among Black SMM is scant and the sample sizes from which existing data are drawn are small. Still, studies generally indicate a significant correlation between self-identified sexual positioning labels, sexual behaviors, and health outcomes among SMM. Specially, SMM who identify as "top" are more likely to report engaging in and have a higher frequency of IAI compared to those who identify as "versatile" or "bottom." Conversely, those who identify as "bottom" are more likely

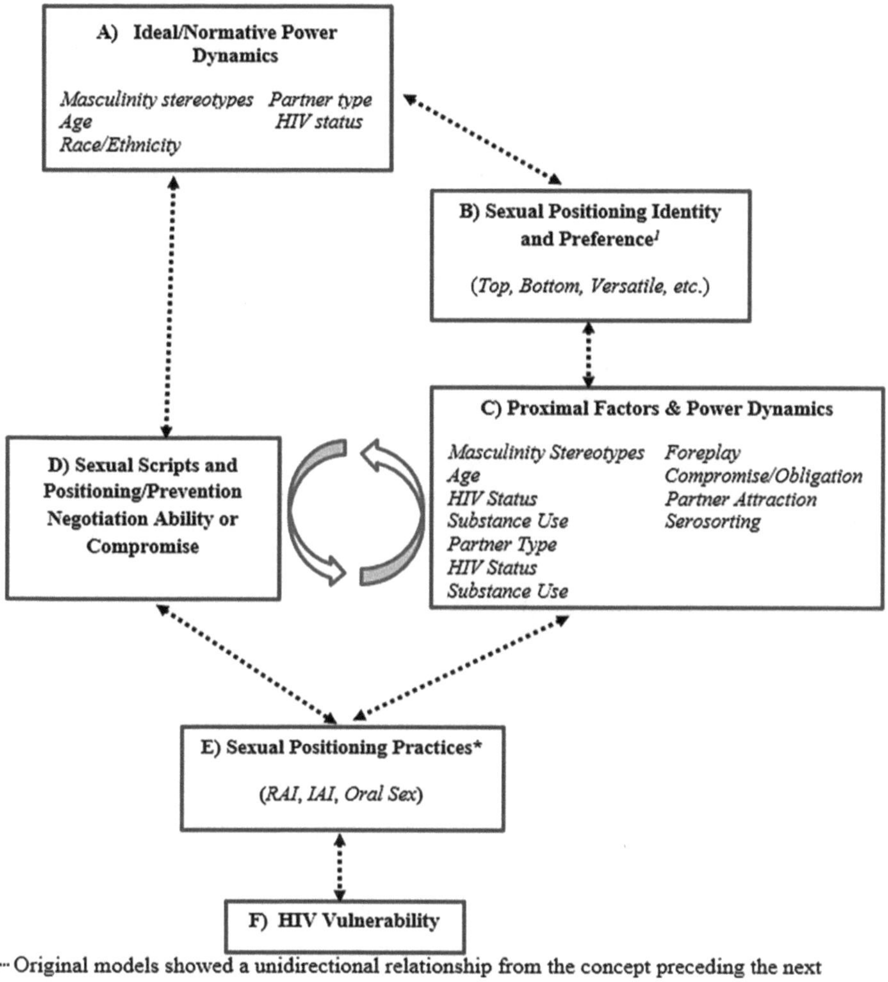

Fig. 1.1 Conceptual model of cultural, behavioral, and social dynamics informing sexual positioning and HIV/STI vulnerability adapted from Dangerfield II et al. (2017b, 2018c)

to engage in and have a higher frequency of RAI than those who identify as "top" or "versatile" (Hart et al., 2003; Moskowitz et al., 2008; Wegesin & Meyer-Bahlburg, 2000; Wei & Raymond, 2010). Men who identify as "versatile" exhibit varying frequencies of both IAI and RAI (Lyons et al., 2011; Shaw et al., 2019; Wei & Raymond, 2010). However, these self-identified roles likely change over the life course and do not necessarily always correlate consistently with actual sexual behaviors (Dangerfield II et al., 2017a; Pachankis et al., 2013). For example, some men who identify as "top" may still engage in RAI while some who identify as "bottom" may occasionally participate in IAI. Studies indicate that IAI is practiced by 32–93% of Black SMM, RAI is reported by 32–50%, and oral sex is 83% prevalent

(Brooks et al., 2015; Harawa et al., 2014; Koblin et al., 2013; Wei & Raymond, 2010). The inconsistency between self-identified sexual role labels and actual sexual behaviors highlights the complexity and fluidity of sexuality within the community. This fluidity underscores the notion that sexual role labels may not always rigidly dictate sexual practices, but rather serve as general indicators of preference that can vary based on individual circumstances, partners, and situational factors (Dangerfield II et al., 2018c).

In light of data showing the diversity of sexual role identification within SMM generally and Black SMM specifically, future research should focus on developing more inclusive frameworks that account for this variation. Additionally, the variability in how men label themselves versus their actual behaviors may also reflect broader social or cultural influences such as stigma, masculinity expectations, or relationship dynamics that shape how these roles are expressed and understood (Dangerfield II et al., 2018c; Fields et al., 2012; Malebranche et al., 2007, 2010). However, despite these critical issues, few studies have focused on these dynamics, highlighting the need for more comprehensive research in this area.

Demographic, Psychosocial, and Behavioral Correlates of Sexual Positioning

Several complex factors play a significant role in shaping sexual epidemiology and related health outcomes for Black SMM (Dangerfield II et al., 2017b, 2018c). Understanding these correlates provides a comprehensive view of the factors that drive sexual behaviors and can inform relevant studies and solutions for the community. Sexual role preferences, such as identifying as top, bottom, or versatile, not only reflect individual sexual identities but also are associated with various behavioral, psychosocial, and cultural factors. These factors, while significant, might not represent an exhaustive list; however, the following draw from the literature to provide valuable insights into the nuanced dynamics among Black SMM to offer a foundation for future studies.

Race

The role of race in sexual epidemiology among Black SMM extends beyond mere statistical representation and delves into the deep-rooted social perceptions and stereotypes that shape sexual identity and behavior. First, Black men are often overrepresented as "tops" than other roles in studies, highlighting either a preference or reporting a social expectation that aligns with longstanding racialized notions of masculinity. This phenomenon can be partly attributed to cultural stereotypes that frame Black men as "masculine" and sexually dominant, reinforcing the expectation that they occupy insertive roles during sexual encounters (Husbands et al., 2013; Malebranche et al., 2007; Wilson et al., 2009). These racialized expectations can influence Black SMM's sexual positioning preferences, their willingness to adopt certain health practices, and their ability to communicate openly with partners (and researchers) about sexual health. Research suggests that perceptions of HIV/STI risk are racialized; Black partners are viewed as riskier and white partners perceived as "safer" (Ober et al., 2018; Wilson et al., 2009). These racist perceptions can shape patterns of partner selection and sexual decision-making. Studies suggest that racial attraction might differ by sexual role among Black SMM (Wade & Nguyễn, 2024; Wilson et al., 2009), which could have implications for HIV/STI epidemiology. The intersection of race (or racism) and sexual positioning preferences highlights harmful stereotypes while perpetuating sexual health inequities. Understanding how race and associated stereotypes influence sexual epidemiology can inform future studies and interventions that challenge harmful stereotypes and support the diverse realities of Black SMM.

Sexual Orientation

Sexual orientation intersects with sexual role preferences in complex ways that remain understudied among SMM groups. For example, studies indicate that men who identify as "gay" or "homosexual" are more likely to report RAI (or "bottoming") than those who identify as "bisexual" (Maulsby et al., 2013; Wheeler et al., 2008). Data highlight nuanced patterns of IAI and RAI among bisexual Black SMM and suggest that these are influenced by various partner dynamics and contextual factors. For example, a latent class analysis of Black bisexual men from 3 U.S. cities showed that men exhibit different probabilities of condomless IAI and RAI based on their partner's HIV status and relationship type (Dangerfield II et al., 2018b). Among the study's latent classes, those in the Seropositive Serosorters group had a high likelihood of engaging in condomless IAI (80.9%) and RAI (67.9%) with main male partners, as well as with non-main male partners living with HIV (70.3% and 60.8%, respectively). Conversely, individuals in the Seronegative/Unknown Serosorters group were more likely to engage in condomless IAI with HIV-negative or status-unknown non-main male partners (59.6%). These findings suggest that sexual positioning among Black bisexual men is influenced not only by sexual orientation but also by contextual factors such as HIV serosorting and partner dynamics. Differential patterns in sexual positioning among bisexual Black SMM by sexual orientation underscore the importance of exploring how personal and social dynamics shape these behaviors and their implications for targeted HIV prevention strategies. These findings demonstrate how sexual positioning practices vary across contexts and partner characteristics, highlighting the need for studies focused on the role of sexual orientation and related positioning practices among Black SMM. However, the dearth of data on bisexual Black SMM means that critical aspects of their sexual health, such as how bisexual identity impacts engagement with healthcare systems or influences HIV prevention strategies, remain underexplored.

Age

Data show that the age of first oral and anal sex among Black SMM is around 14 and 15, respectively (Halkitis et al., 2021). However, the literature focused on age and sexual epidemiology among Black SMM is limited. Overall, studies suggest that age can play a significant role in shaping sexual roles and behaviors among general SMM groups driven by personal growth, relationship dynamics, broader developmental influences, and shifting physical health. For example, data showed that RAI declines with age: 28% of SMM aged 16–29 reported engaging in RAI, compared to 20% of those aged 30–49, and 15% of SMM aged 50 and older. Men over 50 were more likely to report a higher degree of versatility compared to younger age groups (Lyons et al., 2011). Among a sample of men aged 40 and older who have sex with men, those under age 60 were more likely to report RAI compared to those over 60 (Jacobs et al., 2010). Data also show that some SMM change sexual role identity, and subsequently sexual positioning practices, over time (Dangerfield II et al., 2017a; Pachankis et al., 2013). With age, sexual positioning identity and practice can change due to personal growth, experience, confidence, and self-awareness (Dangerfield II et al., 2017a; Pachankis et al., 2013). These shifts might also be influenced by changing physical health, relationship dynamics, and evolving desires for emotional connection as men age. Additionally, social, cultural, and historical contexts can shape these changes, as generational differences in attitudes toward sexuality and societal pressures affect how sexual behaviors and identities are accepted and expressed over time. By recognizing these complex factors regarding age and time, researchers can better understand the nuances of sexual health among Black SMM.

Seropositioning: Sex Based Upon HIV Status

Seropositioning, also referred to as strategic positioning, involves choosing a different sexual position depending on the HIV status of the sexual partner within serodiscordant relationships (i.e., relationships where one partner is living with HIV and the other is HIV-negative). Seropositioning is based on the belief that HIV risk is lessened when "topping" a partner who is living with HIV (Parsons et al., 2006; Van de Ven et al., 2002). Studies suggest that Black SMM are not likely to practice seropositioning (Vallabhaneni et al., 2012; Wei et al., 2010), but data also show that some HIV-negative Black SMM intentionally "top" partners that they know or believe are living with HIV (Dacus et al., 2017; Murphy et al., 2012; Ober et al., 2018; Van de Ven et al., 2002). Similarly, some partners who are living with HIV strategically practice RAI under the belief that it will keep their partners who top them "safer." The protective value of strategic positioning has been widely debated in the literature and the findings of the protective value are mixed (Eaton et al., 2009; Jin et al., 2015; Parsons et al., 2006). Seropositioning and other serosorting behaviors can increase HIV/STI vulnerability relative to consistent condom use because partners may not know their own serostatus and might incorrectly guess the serostatus of their sexual partners (Kennedy et al., 2013; Marks et al., 2010; Vallabhaneni et al., 2012; Zablotska et al., 2009). The inconsistency between attitudes and behaviors toward seropositioning among Black SMM creates an important aspect of risk profiles that need further exploration. Given these risks, prevention scientists must delve deeper into understanding the role of sexual positioning in HIV/STI transmission, including how these behaviors evolve with time and changes in partners. It is also unclear if those who are living with HIV strategically bottom for risk reduction or if bottom behaviors contributed to their initial infection given the associated risks of RAI relative to topping. Research in that area can inform strategies that promote safer practices while recognizing the complexities of sexual decision-making in serodiscordant relationships. Moreover, it is limiting to view the sexual practices of Black gay and bisexual men solely through the lens of risk avoidance and disease prevention. Focusing exclusively on risk reduction can overshadow the broader context of Black SMM's sexual experiences that also encompass aspects of pleasure, intimacy, and emotional connection (Dangerfield II et al., 2017a, 2018c; Moskowitz & Garcia, 2019).

Substance Use

Data show associations between condomless IAI and RAI, binge alcohol use, and recreational drug use among Black SMM (Bruce et al., 2013; Jacobs et al., 2010; Mimiaga et al., 2010; Vosburgh et al., 2012), but few studies have examined how substance use factors into relative sexual positioning practices, especially not among Black SMM. Studies often examine the relationship between substance use and condom use during sex without focusing on how drug or alcohol use affect the likelihood of condomless RAI or IAI. Qualitative data suggest that substance use can influence willingness to accommodate a partner's sexual preferences (Dangerfield II et al., 2017a), often leading individuals to engage in sexual practices they might otherwise avoid. However, the direction of the relationship between personal preferences (including motivations for drug use) and actual sexual practices under the influence of substances remains unclear. This gap highlights the need for more nuanced research on how substance use affect decision-making in sexual positioning, particularly among Black SMM.

Childhood Sexual Abuse

Studies consistently show alarmingly high 23%–40% prevalence of childhood sexual abuse (CSA) among Black SMM (Dangerfield II et al., 2017a; Dharma et al., 2024; Fields et al., 2008; Phillips et al., 2014), which plays a significant and often under-recognized role in shaping sexual behaviors, decision-making, and overall health. The link between CSA and sexual positioning practices is complex and multifaceted. It is well-established that experiencing CSA can have profound and lasting effects on brain development, influencing areas associated with emotional regulation, risk assessment, and impulse control (O'Cleirigh et al., 2012; Relf, 2001). These neurobiological impacts can contribute to altered decision-making processes including impulsivity, heightened risk-taking, and difficulties in establishing boundaries, which can manifest in adulthood as increased vulnerability to high-risk sexual behaviors. For Black SMM, these behaviors can include a greater likelihood of engaging in condomless sex (Lloyd & Operario, 2012; Mimiaga et al., 2009). Some studies suggest that individuals with a history of CSA may be more inclined to engage in RAI (which confers greater risk of HIV acquisition than IAI) due to psychological factors such as diminished self-worth, a perceived need to please partners, or a pattern of reenacting traumatic experiences to process or normalize them. This can lead to patterns where the individual may prioritize partner satisfaction over their own safety (Dangerfield II et al., 2017a), impacting condom use behaviors. The trauma from CSA can also lead to a higher likelihood of substance use as a coping mechanism, further increasing HIV/STI risk. Addressing the impacts of CSA within the context of sexual epidemiology is essential for developing trauma-informed and holistic public health interventions that prioritize mental health support, foster resilience, and promote safer sexual practices.

Sexual Health Behaviors

Data increasingly suggests that some health behaviors such as PrEP use, HIV testing, and rectal douching might be associated with sexual roles among Black SMM. For example, those who identify as "bottom" or "versatile" engaged more frequently in practices like rectal douching or enema use compared to those who identify as "top" (Dangerfield II et al., 2020). Additionally, Black SMM who "bottom" are more likely than not to have greater perceived risk for HIV and PrEP interest (Dangerfield II & Anderson, 2024). Sexual roles could influence broader health outcomes such as mental health and quality of life. For example, bottoms, who might feel more vulnerable due to their perceived higher risk of HIV exposure, may experience increased anxiety and stress related to sexual encounters (Dacus et al., 2017). These psychological factors can contribute to reduced sexual satisfaction and potentially affect relationship dynamics, leading to increased tension or dissatisfaction in their sexual and romantic lives.

The varied perceived vulnerability according to sexual roles is a key understudied cultural factor in the sexual epidemiology of SMM groups generally and even more crucial for health promotion among Black SMM. The cultural connotations associated with these roles can reinforce certain behaviors and expectations among SMM. For example, tops may feel pressure to assert dominance or exhibit traditionally masculine traits, which could affect their willingness to seek regular health check-ups or openly discuss their sexual health with partners and healthcare providers. On the other hand, bottoms may experience stigma or internalized shame, which could discourage them from engaging in proactive sexual health behaviors, such as routine STI testing or disclosing their sexual role to clinicians. The psychosocial and behavioral differences highlight the need for targeted sexual health interventions that address the unique risks and preventative strategies associated with each sexual role. Although health behaviors are often tied to role preferences, the implications extend beyond individual choice to cultural norms and access to health resources. This highlights the importance of culturally competent public health approaches that acknowledge and address the unique behaviors and motivations within Black SMM communities.

Cultural Dynamics and Sexual Epidemiology

Gendered Sexual Roles

We previously discussed how power dynamics and based upon gender roles in heterosexual partnerships can create disparities in decision-making power around sexual practices and condom use to according to the Theory of Gender and Power (Connell, 2014; Wingood & DiClemente, 2000). As previously suggested, Black SMM often navigate societal and community expectations of masculinity that manifest in their relationships and influence sexual epidemiology and health. For example, within some same-sex relationships, sexual positioning is "gendered" by a top and bottom relational dynamic (Dangerfield et al. 2017a; Hoppe, 2011; Johns et al., 2012; Moskowitz & Garcia, 2019). Some SMM who identify as "bottoms" or receptive partners may assume the role of a "woman" (as described by SMM) within relationships, accept sexual vulnerability which could include condomless sex (Dangerfield et al. 2017a; Hoppe, 2011; Johns et al., 2012). The expectations regarding gender and power are complicated by a same-sex dynamic in which both partners are "men." For Black SMM, top and bottom dynamics are compounded by the racialized stereotypes that frame them as masculine, dominant, and reinforce expectations for them to be "tops" (Fields et al., 2012; Husbands et al., 2013; Malebranche & Bryant, 2005). Some SMM use versatility to redistribute power within the dynamic or reject heterosexual norms; contemporary data show increased proportions of samples reporting identifying as "versatile" than other categories.

The cultural expectation for Black SMM to be "tops" creates a unique conundrum that affects their identity, relationship dynamics, and sexual health. For example, cultural expectations can pressure them to conform to desired sexual roles even if it conflicts with their personal preferences or comfort. This pressure can limit authentic self-expression and contribute to a constrained view of their sexual roles. This expectation can also lead to challenges in negotiating safer sex practices, as

Black SMM who are perceived as "tops" might face the responsibility for condom use (along with other "manly" duties in a relationship) being automatically assigned to them, regardless of their actual desires or negotiation capacity. On one hand, the societal perception of being a "top" could shield them from the stigma associated with being a "bottom," but it can simultaneously expose them to stereotypes that strip away their agency and reduce their identity to one-dimensional characteristics of dominance and power. The need to adhere to these roles to meet societal or partner expectations might conflict with their genuine sexual preferences, leading to internalized stigma and stress. Versatility, where roles are interchangeable, offers a path for some partners to share power and mutual decision-making within relationships (Dangerfield II et al., 2017b; Dworkin et al., 2017), but the internal and external pressures related to positioning and perceived power dynamics require further attention and study. Recognizing and addressing these expectations is crucial for fostering healthier relationship dynamics and improving quality of life for the community.

Religiosity and Spirituality

Religiosity and spirituality are salient cultural aspects of identity that can significantly influence the beliefs, behaviors, and decision-making processes of communities across populations. This influence includes sexual epidemiology, and even more specifically, sexual positioning among Black SMM (Dangerfield II et al., 2019; Jeffries et al., 2008). Religion often plays a dual role—providing community support and moral guidance, while also potentially reinforcing stigma and restrictive norms around sexuality. For Black SMM, whose cultural and community ties may be intertwined with religious practices, these influences can lead to internal conflicts regarding sexual expression and role preferences and can impact sexual epidemiology. Spirituality—distinct from organized religion—might offer more personalized frameworks that allow for reconciling sexual identity with personal beliefs, potentially influencing how individuals approach sexual roles and their comfort with discussing or exploring different practices (Dangerfield II et al., 2019). Increasingly, Black SMM are adopting "spirituality" as a way to reconcile conflicts between their religious upbringing and sexual identity, distancing themselves from rigid religious structures. This shift often liberates them to explore their sexuality more freely, which can encourage both safe practices grounded in self-worth and, conversely, sexual behaviors with fewer psychological constraints. Black SMM qualitatively reported bottoming as a deeply personal and selective act tied to spiritual connection and trust (Dangerfield II et al., 2019). However, while religiosity and spirituality affect partner selection and sexual roles, they do not consistently mediate condom use. While studies have touched on the broader impacts of religion and spirituality on sexual health and behaviors for Black SMM (Foster et al., 2011; Jeffries IV et al., 2017; Jeffries et al., 2008), there is a notable gap specifically examining how these factors shape sexual positioning practices among Black SMM. The need to further explore these dynamics includes clarifying how religious and spiritual frameworks impact sexual decision-making, particularly in the context of HIV prevention and broader health behaviors.

Partner Dynamics

Within partner dynamics, key factors such as attraction, intimacy, compromise, and obligation play significant roles in shaping sexual positioning practices among Black SMM. Attraction often drives initial sexual behaviors, but deeper emotional intimacy within a relationship can lead individuals to adapt their sexual roles to align with their partner's preferences or expectations, even when these do not match their typical preferences (Dangerfield II et al., 2017a, 2018c). This adaptability reflects a desire to enhance emotional connection, maintain relationship harmony, or ensure their partner's satisfaction, emphasizing the emotional significance tied to sexual positioning practices. For many, sexual roles extend beyond physical desires, becoming a reflection of relational dynamics and emotional bonds.

As intimacy deepens, sexual positioning can evolve to reflect greater openness and fluidity, driven by a desire for deeper emotional connections and mutual understanding within the partnership (Dangerfield II et al., 2017a; Pachankis et al., 2013). Romantic relationships, as opposed to casual encounters, are more likely to elicit this adaptability, as emotional investment reshapes typical sexual behavior patterns (Dangerfield II et al., 2017a). Over time, emotional satisfaction can take precedence alongside physical pleasure, prompting shifts in sexual roles to meet the evolving needs of the relationship (Hoppe, 2011; Johns et al., 2012). This fluidity enables Black SMM to move away from rigid sexual roles, fostering more diverse experiences that align with their partner's and their emotional and physical desires.

Compromise and obligation are influential relationship factors, as individuals may adjust their behaviors to meet a partner's expectations or avoid conflict, sometimes at the expense of their personal preferences or health-related priorities. These dynamics can affect decisions around condom use and engagement in HIV prevention strategies such as PrEP, potentially increasing health vulnerabilities when negotiation power is reduced (Dangerfield II et al., 2018c). The interplay of attraction, intimacy, compromise, and obligation highlights how sexual positioning is deeply relational, shaped by emotional bonds and power dynamics within partnerships. By integrating more of these relational factors, a more comprehensive understanding of sexual health behaviors and identity development among Black SMM can be achieved, particularly as they intersect with race, age, and sexual orientation.

Sexual Epidemiology and Health Outcomes

The consequences of sexual positioning practices among Black SMM are multifaceted, impacting physical health, mental health, and social experiences. The preference for or adoption of certain sexual roles can expose individuals to different health risks and the psychological impacts of these dynamics can lead to stress, reduced self-esteem, and internalized stigma, further complicating efforts to maintain and promote health behaviors. Public health initiatives must consider these varied consequences to design targeted, supportive interventions that resonate with Black SMM.

HIV and Other STIs

Probably the most apparent health implication of sexual roles and related positioning is the relative risks for HIV and STIs. Men who practice condomless RAI (bottom) with male partners are statistically more likely to acquire HIV and rectal STIs than men who only participate in condomless IAI (or top) (Baggaley et al., 2010, 2018; Vittinghoff et al., 1999). Both RAI and IAI can facilitate HIV acquisition and transmission. Condomless RAI allows HIV easier access to the bloodstream due to the thin rectal lining and increased risk of tearing during sex. Similarly, condomless IAI increases the risk of HIV entering through the opening of the penis. Versatility (practicing both IAI and RAI) for anal sexual positioning thus increases the chance of infection and transmission to sexual partners (Dangerfield II et al., 2017b; Lyons et al., 2011; Shaw et al., 2019; van Druten et al., 1992). In other words, men who practice both "top" (i.e., insertive) and "bottom" (i.e., receptive) roles for anal sex may be at high risk for HIV and STI infection via RAI and can potentiate subsequent risk for HIV and STIs to male partners through IAI. Oral sex confers risk for extragenital STIs, which facilitate drug resistant bacteria (Bissessor et al., 2014; Edwards & Carne, 1998; Unemo & Nicholas, 2012). The variations of sexual positioning practices can create different risk profiles among men who have sex with men and the broader population (Dangerfield II et al., 2017b, 2018b; Wilken et al., 2016). Some men might practice RAI and IAI within the same sexual encounter with the same partner, practice RAI and IAI in different sexual acts with the same partner, or practice RAI with some male partners and IAI with others (Dangerfield II et al., 2017a, 2017b; Wilken et al., 2016). Therefore, it is important to understand the contexts for a given sexual encounter as SMM may not simply practice just RAI or IAI in one encounter. Rather, there could also be a wider range of contextual "top" and "bottom" practices with certain partners over others, leading to an understudied range of versatility practice (and associated health outcomes). Moreover, bisexual men who engage in versatility with male partners can also increased risk of transmitting HIV/STIs to their female partners (Dangerfield II et al., 2018a; Malebranche et al., 2010; Wilken et al., 2016). The ability to transmit and acquire infections across different sexual networks highlights the importance of targeted efforts that study and address the unique risks associated with sexual positioning.

Stigma and Mental Health

Unaddressed sexual epidemiology among Black SMM can have significant consequences, contributing to internalized stigma and anal sex stigma that negatively impact health and quality of life. When the specific sexual health needs and realities of Black SMM are overlooked, misconceptions and stereotypes are allowed to persist, reinforcing stigmas related to sexual roles and practices, such as bottoming (Winder, 2023; Ober et al., 2018). This stigma can lead to shame and reluctance to disclose sexual practices to healthcare providers, hindering access to preventive measures like PrEP and comprehensive STI screening. Internalized stigma can erode self-esteem and mental health, increasing feelings of isolation and reducing the likelihood of engaging in open conversations about sexual health with partners and clinicians. The compounded effects of this stigma contribute to poorer health outcomes and can perpetuate cycles of high-risk behavior due to a lack of supportive and affirming care. The significance of addressing these stigmas extends beyond physical health to overall health and quality of life. Internalized anal sex stigma can affect psychological distress that impacts daily functioning, relationship dynamics, and willingness to seek medical attention. This can result in delayed diagnoses, reduced treatment adherence, and a general hesitancy to engage with healthcare systems. Public health approaches that focus on culturally responsive education and de-stigmatization efforts are essential for fostering a supportive environment that empowers Black SMM. Addressing sexuality stigma and promoting positive sexual health narratives can help improve health outcomes, enhance mental well-being, and ensure that Black SMM have equitable opportunities for a healthy, fulfilling life.

Cancer

Oral and anal cancers, which are linked to persistent human papillomavirus (HPV) infection, are an important yet often overlooked consequence of sexual epidemiology among Black SMM. Despite the established connection between HPV and anal cancer, there is limited research specifically addressing how sexual positioning practices affects the prevalence of anal cancer among Black SMM, particularly among those who bottom. This oversight is significant due to disparities in healthcare access, lower rates of HPV vaccination, and infrequent anal Pap smears, all compounded by stigma that deters individuals from seeking preventive care. Current sexual epidemiology research tends to focus on HIV and other non-HPV STIs, leaving a critical gap in understanding and addressing anal cancer risks. Expanding research to include anal cancer and implementing culturally competent outreach can help identify specific risk factors and promote prevention strategies, ensuring Black SMM receive comprehensive sexual health care.

Conclusions and Recommendations for Prevention Science and Service Research

The complex dynamics of sexual epidemiology among Black SMM underscores the need for more in-depth research to better understand the factors influencing HIV/STI incidence. Overall, sexual epidemiology is contextual and influenced by a range of factors that are affected and can affect dynamics within the community and between partners. Recognizing the complex interplay between sexual role labels, sexual behaviors, and broader health outcomes is crucial for designing effective public health strategies. However, despite the importance of these dynamics, there remains a lack of comprehensive and reliable measures for assessing sexual positioning in sexual epidemiology and prevention science, limiting the ability to fully understand and address the nuances of sexual behavior and health outcomes among diverse SMM populations. Advancing research and developing better measures to study these complexities is essential for creating more effective interventions. Standardizing measures to assess the relationship between self-identified sexual roles and actual sexual positioning practices are crucial, as is exploring how these practices evolve throughout the life course. Without robust measures, efforts to provide relevant sexual health services for diverse SMM subgroups may fall short, reinforcing existing disparities rather than reducing them.

Future studies should focus on how social, psychological, and demographic factors—including age, race, risk perceptions, and health beliefs—affect sexual behavior and health among Black SMM. Longitudinal research would be particularly valuable in tracking how sexual positioning behaviors change over time and how these changes impact health outcomes, offering a more comprehensive understanding of the factors contributing to sexual health disparities. It is also essential to consider the unique experiences of bisexual men, whose risk perceptions and condom use practices may vary depending on the gender of their partners, potentially creating different transmission dynamics. Attention should also be paid to the distinct power dynamics and sexual decision-making processes within various gay/queer subgroups, such as those in the house/ballroom or non-binary, communities, which may shape sexual behavior in ways that differ from broader populations. Understanding these diverse factors can enhance public health strategies by providing a more nuanced view of sexual health behaviors across different subgroups.

Interventions that account for these nuances and provide tailored, stigma-free support for SMM across different sexual roles are still needed. Tailored approaches that acknowledge these variations could enhance the effectiveness of public health strategies, improving outcomes by addressing the specific concerns and behaviors of tops, bottoms, and versatile individuals, among others. Moreover, interventions that consider the fluidity and complexity of sexual role identities could better support those whose behaviors may not consistently align with their self-identified roles, thereby reducing the overall risk of HIV and other STIs within the MSM community.

One key area for intervention development is enhancing access to culturally competent healthcare. Black SMM often face barriers related to stigma, shame, and economic challenges that impede their ability to access PrEP, regular STI screening, and comprehensive health education. Interventions that prioritize cultural competence in healthcare settings, ensuring providers are trained to understand and respect the unique experiences of Black SMM, can help mitigate these challenges. Clinicians and researchers must be equipped with the knowledge to address the unique needs of SMM, which includes training clinicians to improve communication and reduce stigma in medical settings. Additionally, creating targeted outreach and education campaigns that resonate with the specific cultural and social norms within Black SMM communities can promote better engagement with prevention activities and health services (Habarta et al., 2017). Ultimately, effective interventions must go beyond addressing individual behaviors to tackle the broader societal and systemic determinants affecting sexual health among Black SMM. Legal protections, anti-discrimination policies, and community-level initiatives that challenge stigmatizing narratives are crucial for fostering environments where Black SMM can openly discuss and manage their sexual health. Combining these comprehensive, theory-based approaches with targeted support across different life stages can promote more equitable health outcomes, reduce disparities, and empower Black SMM to lead healthier, more informed lives. Expanding research in these areas will not only deepen our understanding of sexual epidemiology among SMM but also contribute to reducing health disparities and fostering greater equity in sexual health outcomes.

Raised Questions

1. What role does sexual epidemiology play in the differences in sexual health outcomes observed among SMM?
2. What statistical models and other research methodologies are best suited to study sexual epidemiology among Black SMM?
3. What are the best measures to study the role of sexual positioning practices among SMM?

Chapter Summary

This chapter explored the complex dynamics of sexual epidemiology among Black sexual SMM and emphasized the need for more comprehensive research to design more holist interventions. It highlighted gaps in understanding sexual positioning, roles, and their impact on HIV/STI vulnerability, especially across different ethnic groups and subcultures. Future research should focus on how social, psychological, and demographic factors influence sexual epidemiology, with an emphasis on tailored, culturally sensitive interventions. Standardized measures and more research on sexual positioning practices across the life course are also crucial for advancing the study of sexual epidemiology within prevention science.

Key Points

1. **Conceptualizing sexual epidemiology**: Sexual epidemiology is introduced as a field of study that examines the distribution, patterns, and determinants of sexual behavior within populations. It highlights the need for more comprehensive research into sexual behaviors and their connection to health outcomes, particularly among Black SMM. This field helps understand behavioral and cultural dynamics and inform sexual health interventions.
2. **The role of sexual positioning practices on health outcomes**: Sexual positioning practices (insertive or receptive anal sex roles) play a critical role in HIV/STI vulnerability among SMM. Research shows that men who practice receptive anal intercourse (RAI) are at a higher risk for HIV/STIs than those who only engage in insertive anal intercourse (IAI). The complexity of sexual positioning practices, including versatility (engaging in both roles), should be further explored to understand behavioral and cultural dynamics, risk profiles, and prevention strategies.
3. **The Influence of cultural, psychological, and social dynamics on sexual behavior**: Cultural perceptions of gender, power, and race influence sexual behaviors and partner preferences among Black SMM. These factors shape sexual positioning practices, which can affect HIV/STI vulnerability. The chapter emphasizes the importance of considering the broader social and relational dynamics in sexual health interventions.
4. **The fluidity and complexity of sexual roles**: Sexual role identities (e.g., top, bottom, versatile) are not always fixed and can evolve over time due to personal growth, changes in relationships, and shifting interests for emotional connection. This fluidity underscores the need for nuanced approaches to sexual health education, risk reduction, and clinical interventions that reflect the diversity of sexual preferences and experiences among Black SMM.
5. **Scientific gaps and methodological challenges**: There is a lack of consistent measures and thorough research on sexual positioning practices, the role of age in sexual development, and the need for standardized methodologies to study sexual epidemiology among Black SMM.

References

Anderson, R. M. (2013). Positive sexuality and its impact on overall well-being. *Bundesgesundheitsblatt - Gesundheitsforschung - Gesundheitsschutz, 56*(2), 208–214. https://doi.org/10.1007/s00103-012-1607-z

Baggaley, R. F., White, R. G., & Boily, M.-C. (2010). HIV transmission risk through anal intercourse: Systematic review, meta-analysis and implications for HIV prevention. *International Journal of Epidemiology, dyq057*. https://doi.org/10.1093/ije/dyq057

Baggaley, R. F., Owen, B. N., Silhol, R., Elmes, J., Anton, P., McGowan, I., van der Straten, A., Shacklett, B., Dang, Q., Swann, E. M., Bolton, D. L., & Boily, M.-C. (2018). Does per-act HIV-1 transmission risk through anal sex vary by gender? An updated systematic review and meta-analysis. *American Journal of Reproductive Immunology, 0*(0), e13039. https://doi.org/10.1111/aji.13039

Beyrer, C., Sullivan, P. S., Sanchez, J., Dowdy, D., Altman, D., Trapence, G., Collins, C., Katabira, E., Kazatchkine, M., Sidibe, M., & Mayer, K. H. (2012). A call to action for comprehensive HIV services for men who have sex with men. *The Lancet, 380*(9839), 424–438. https://doi.org/10.1016/S0140-6736(12)61022-8

Bissessor, M., Whiley, D. M., Fairley, C. K., Bradshaw, C. S., Lee, D. M., Snow, A. S., Lahra, M. M., Hocking, J. S., & Chen, M. Y. (2014). Persistence of Neisseria gonorrhoeae DNA following treatment for pharyngeal and rectal gonorrhea is influenced by antibiotic susceptibility and reinfection. *Clinical Infectious Diseases, ciu873*. https://doi.org/10.1093/cid/ciu873

Bond, J. C., & Ford, J. V. (2024). A call for sex-positive epidemiology. *American Journal of Epidemiology, kwae054*. https://doi.org/10.1093/aje/kwae054

Brooks, R. A., Landovitz, R. J., Regan, R., Lee, S.-J., & Allen, V. C. (2015). Perceptions of and intentions to adopt HIV pre-exposure prophylaxis among black men who have sex with men in Los Angeles. *International Journal of STD & AIDS, 26*(14), 1040–1048. https://doi.org/10.1177/0956462415570159

Bruce, D., Kahana, S., Harper, G. W., Fernández, M. I., & ATN, the. (2013). Alcohol use predicts sexual risk behavior with HIV-negative or partners of unknown status among young HIV-positive men who have sex with men. *AIDS Care, 25*(5), 559–565. https://doi.org/10.1080/09540121.2012.720363

Centers for Disease Control and Prevention. (2020, January 27). *Brief | African American | Gay and Bisexual Men | HIV by Group | HIV/AIDS | CDC*. https://www.cdc.gov/hiv/group/msm/brief.html

Connell, R. W. (2014). *Gender and power: Society, the person and sexual politics*. Wiley.

Dacus, J., Voisin, D. R., & Barker, J. (2017). "Proud I Am Negative": Maintaining HIV-seronegativity among Black MSM in New York City. *Men and Masculinities*, 1097184X17696174. https://doi.org/10.1177/1097184X17696174

Dangerfield II, D. (2024, January 18). The significance of sexual epidemiology. *PRIISE: Thought Pieces*. https://priiselab.com/article/the-significance-of-sexual-epidemiology/

Dangerfield, D. T., II, & Anderson, J. N. (2024). A scripted, PrEP-using peer change agent improves perceived risk for HIV and willingness to accept referrals quickly among Black sexual minority men: Preliminary findings from POSSIBLE. *AIDS and Behavior*. https://doi.org/10.1007/s10461-024-04313-2

Dangerfield, D. T., II, Smith, L. R., Anderson, J. N., Bruce, O. J., Farley, J., & Bluthenthal, R. (2017a). Sexual positioning practices and sexual risk among Black gay and bisexual men: A life course perspective. *AIDS and Behavior, 22*(6), 1919–1931. https://doi.org/10.1007/s10461-017-1948-6

Dangerfield, D. T., II, Smith, L. R., Williams, J., Unger, J., & Bluthenthal, R. (2017b). Sexual positioning among men who have sex with men: A narrative review. *Archives of Sexual Behavior, 46*(4), 869–884. https://doi.org/10.1007/s10508-016-0738-y

Dangerfield, D. T., II, Carmack, C. C., Gilreath, T. D., & Duncan, D. T. (2018a). Latent classes of sexual positioning practices and sexual risk among men who have sex with men in Paris, France. *AIDS and Behavior, 22*(12), 4001–4008. https://doi.org/10.1007/s10461-018-2267-2

Dangerfield, D. T., II, Harawa, N. T., Smith, L. R., Jeffries, W. L., Baezconde-Garbanati, L., & Bluthenthal, R. (2018b). Latent classes of sexual risk among Black men who have sex with men and women. *Archives of Sexual Behavior, 47*(7), 2071–2080. https://doi.org/10.1007/s10508-017-1142-y

Dangerfield, D. T., II, Ober, A. J., Smith, L. R., Shoptaw, S., & Bluthenthal, R. N. (2018c). Exploring and adapting a conceptual model of sexual positioning practices and sexual risk among HIV-negative Black men who have sex with men. *The Journal of Sex Research, 55*(8), 1022–1032. https://doi.org/10.1080/00224499.2018.1433287

Dangerfield, D. T., II, Williams, J. E., Bass, A. S., Wynter, T., & Bluthenthal, R. N. (2019). Exploring religiosity and spirituality in the sexual decision-making of black gay and bisexual men. *Journal of Religion and Health, 58*(5), 1792–1802. https://doi.org/10.1007/s10943-019-00845-3

Dangerfield, D. T., II, Johnson, D., Hamlin-Palmer, S., Browne, D. C., Mayer, K. H., & Hickson, D. A. (2020). Prevalence and correlates of rectal douching and enema use among Black sexual minority men and Black transwomen in the Deep South. *Archives of Sexual Behavior.* https://doi.org/10.1007/s10508-019-01605-w

Dharma, C., Keyes, K. M., Rudolph, K. E., Shrader, C.-H., Chen, Y.-T., Schneider, J., & Duncan, D. T. (2024). Adverse childhood experiences among Black sexually minoritized men and Black transgender women in Chicago. *International Journal for Equity in Health, 23*(1), 74. https://doi.org/10.1186/s12939-024-02168-6

Dworkin, S. L., Zakaras, J. M., Campbell, C., Wilson, P., Grisham, K., Chakravarty, D., Neilands, T. B., & Hoff, C. (2017). Relationship power among same-sex male couples in New York and San Francisco: Laying the groundwork for sexual risk reduction interventions focused on interpersonal power. *The Journal of Sex Research, 0*(0), 1–13. https://doi.org/10.1080/00224499.2017.1279258

Eaton, L. A., Kalichman, S. C., O'Connell, D. A., & Karchner, W. D. (2009). A strategy for selecting sexual partners believed to pose little/no risks for HIV: Serosorting and its implications for HIV transmission. *AIDS Care, 21*(10), 1279–1288. https://doi.org/10.1080/09540120902803208

Edwards, S., & Carne, C. (1998). Oral sex and the transmission of viral STIs. *Sexually Transmitted Infections, 74*(1), 6–10. https://doi.org/10.1136/sti.74.1.6

Elopre, L., Ott, C., Lambert, C. C., Amico, K. R., Sullivan, P. S., Marrazzo, J., Mugavero, M. J., & Turan, J. M. (2021). Missed prevention opportunities: Why young, Black MSM with recent HIV diagnosis did not access HIV pre-exposure prophylaxis services. *AIDS and Behavior, 25*(5), 1464–1473. https://doi.org/10.1007/s10461-020-02985-0

Fields, S. D., Malebranche, D., & Feist-Price, S. (2008). Childhood sexual abuse in black men who have sex with men: Results from three qualitative studies. *Cultural Diversity and Ethnic Minority Psychology, 14*(4), 385–390. https://doi.org/10.1037/1099-9809.14.4.385

Fields, E. L., Bogart, L. M., Smith, K. C., Malebranche, D. J., Ellen, J., & Schuster, M. A. (2012). HIV risk and perceptions of masculinity among young Black men who have sex with men. *Journal of Adolescent Health, 50*(3), 296–303. https://doi.org/10.1016/j.jadohealth.2011.07.007

Foster, M. L., Arnold, E., Rebchook, G., & Kegeles, S. M. (2011). 'It's my inner strength': Spirituality, religion and HIV in the lives of young African American men who have sex with men. *Culture, Health & Sexuality, 13*(9), 1103–1117. https://doi.org/10.1080/13691058.2011.600460

Habarta, N., Boudewyns, V., Badal, H., Johnston, J., Uhrig, J., Green, D., Ruddle, P., Rosenthal, J., & Stryker, J. E. (2017). CDC'S testing makes us stronger (TMUS) campaign: Was campaign exposure associated with HIV testing behavior among black gay and bisexual men? *AIDS Education and Prevention, 29*(3), 228–240.

Halkitis, P. N., LoSchiavo, C., Martino, R. J., De La Cruz, B. M., Stults, C. B., & Krause, K. D. (2021). Age of sexual Debut among young gay-identified sexual minority men: The P18 Cohort study. *The Journal of Sex Research, 58*(5), 573–580. https://doi.org/10.1080/00224499.2020.1783505

Harawa, N., Wilton, L., Wang, L., Mao, C., Kuo, I., Penniman, T., Shoptaw, S., Griffith, S., Williams, J. K., Cummings, V., Mayer, K., Koblin, B., & HPTN 061. (2014). Types of female partners reported by Black men who have sex with men and women (MSMW) and associations with intercourse frequency, unprotected sex and HIV and STI prevalence. *AIDS and Behavior, 18*(8), 1548–1559. https://doi.org/10.1007/s10461-014-0704-4

Hart, T. A., Wolitski, R. J., Purcell, D. W., Gómez, C., Halkitis, P., & Team, T. S. U. M. S. (2003). Sexual behavior among HIV-positive men who have sex with men: What's in a label? *The Journal of Sex Research, 40*(2), 179–188. https://doi.org/10.1080/00224490309552179

Hoppe, T. (2011). Circuits of power, circuits of pleasure: Sexual scripting in gay men's bottom narratives. *Sexualities, 14*(2), 193–217. https://doi.org/10.1177/1363460711399033

Husbands, W., Makoroka, L., Walcott, R., Adam, B. D., George, C., Remis, R. S., & Rourke, S. B. (2013). Black gay men as sexual subjects: Race, racialisation and the social relations of sex among Black gay men in Toronto. *Culture, Health & Sexuality, 15*(4), 434–449. https://doi.org/10.1080/13691058.2012.763186

Jacobs, R. J., Fernandez, M. I., Ownby, R. L., Bowen, G. S., Hardigan, P. C., & Kane, M. N. (2010). Factors associated with risk for unprotected receptive and insertive anal intercourse in men aged 40 and older who have sex with men. *AIDS Care, 22*(10), 1204–1211. https://doi.org/10.1080/09540121003615137

Jeffries, W. L. J., IV, Sutton, M. Y., & Eke, A. N. (2017). On the battlefield: The Black church, public health, and the fight against HIV among African American gay and bisexual men. *Journal of Urban Health, 94*(3), 384–398. https://doi.org/10.1007/s11524-017-0147-0

Jeffries, W. L., Dodge, B., & Sandfort, T. G. M. (2008). Religion and spirituality among bisexual Black men in the USA. *Culture, Health & Sexuality, 10*(5), 463–477. https://doi.org/10.1080/13691050701877526

Jin, F., Prestage, G. P., Mao, L., Poynten, I. M., Templeton, D. J., Grulich, A. E., & Zablotska, I. (2015). "Any condomless anal intercourse" is no longer an accurate measure of HIV sexual risk behavior in gay and other men who have sex with men. *Frontiers in Immunology, 6*. https://doi.org/10.3389/fimmu.2015.00086

Johns, M. M., Pingel, E., Eisenberg, A., Santana, M. L., & Bauermeister, J. (2012). Butch tops and femme bottoms? Sexual positioning, sexual decision making, and gender roles among young gay men. *American Journal of Men's Health, 6*(6), 505–518. https://doi.org/10.1177/1557988312455214

Kennedy, C. E., Bernard, L. J., Muessig, K. E., Konda, K. A., Akl, E. A., Lo, Y.-R., Gerbase, A., & O'Reilly, K. R. (2013). Serosorting and HIV/STI infection among HIV-negative MSM and transgender people: A systematic review and meta-analysis to inform WHO guidelines. *Journal of Sexually Transmitted Diseases, 2013*, e583627. https://doi.org/10.1155/2013/583627

Koblin, B. A., Mayer, K. H., Eshleman, S. H., Wang, L., Mannheimer, S., del Rio, C., Shoptaw, S., Magnus, M., Buchbinder, S., Wilton, L., Liu, T.-Y., Cummings, V., Piwowar-Manning, E., Fields, S. D., Griffith, S., Elharrar, V., & Wheeler, D. (2013). Correlates of HIV acquisition in a cohort of Black men who have sex with men in the United States: HIV Prevention Trials Network (HPTN) 061. *PLoS ONE, 8*(7), e70413. https://doi.org/10.1371/journal.pone.0070413

Lefkowitz, E. S., & Vasilenko, S. A. (2014). Healthy sex and sexual health: New directions for studying outcomes of sexual health. *New Directions for Child and Adolescent Development, 2014*(144), 87–98. https://doi.org/10.1002/cad.20062

Lloyd, S., & Operario, D. (2012). HIV risk among men who have sex with men who have experienced childhood sexual abuse: Systematic review and meta-analysis. *AIDS Education and Prevention, 24*(3), 228–241. https://doi.org/10.1521/aeap.2012.24.3.228

Lyons, A., Pitts, M., Smith, G., Grierson, J., Smith, A., McNally, S., & Couch, M. (2011). Versatility and HIV vulnerability: Investigating the proportion of Australian gay men having both insertive and receptive anal intercourse. *The Journal of Sexual Medicine, 8*(8), 2164–2171. https://doi.org/10.1111/j.1743-6109.2010.02197.x

Malebranche, D. J., & Bryant, L. (2005). *Masclulinity & HIV risk among black MSM*. National HIV Prevention Conference, Atlanta, GA.

Malebranche, D. J., Fields, E. L., Bryant, L. O., & Harper, S. R. (2007). Masculine socialization and sexual risk behaviors among Black men who have sex with men: A qualitative exploration. *Men and Masculinities*. https://doi.org/10.1177/1097184X07309504

Malebranche, D. J., Arriola, K. J., Jenkins, T. R., Dauria, E., & Patel, S. N. (2010). Exploring the "Bisexual Bridge": A qualitative study of risk behavior and disclosure of same-sex behavior among Black bisexual men. *American Journal of Public Health, 100*(1), 159–164. https://doi.org/10.2105/AJPH.2008.158725

Marks, G., Millett, G. A., Bingham, T., Lauby, J., Murrill, C. S., & Stueve, A. (2010). Prevalence and protective value of serosorting and strategic positioning among Black and Latino men who have sex with men. *Sexually Transmitted Diseases, 37*(5), 325. https://doi.org/10.1097/OLQ.0b013e3181c95dac

Maulsby, C., Millett, G., Lindsey, K., Kelley, R., Johnson, K., Montoya, D., & Holtgrave, D. (2013). HIV among Black men who have sex with men (MSM) in the United States: A review of the literature. *AIDS and Behavior, 18*(1), 10–25. https://doi.org/10.1007/s10461-013-0476-2

Mimiaga, M. J., Noonan, E., Donnell, D., Safren, S. A., Koenen, K. C., Gortmaker, S., O'Cleirigh, C., Chesney, M. A., Coates, T. J., Koblin, B. A., & Mayer, K. H. (2009). Childhood sexual abuse is highly associated with HIV risk–taking behavior and infection among MSM in the EXPLORE Study. *Journal of Acquired Immune Deficiency Syndromes (1999), 51*(3), 340–348. https://doi.org/10.1097/QAI.0b013e3181a24b38

Mimiaga, M. J., Reisner, S. L., Fontaine, Y.-M., Bland, S. E., Driscoll, M. A., Isenberg, D., Cranston, K., Skeer, M. R., & Mayer, K. H. (2010). Walking the line: Stimulant use during sex and HIV risk behavior among Black urban MSM. *Drug and Alcohol Dependence, 110*(1), 30–37. https://doi.org/10.1016/j.drugalcdep.2010.01.017

Moskowitz, D. A., & Garcia, C. P. (2019). Top, bottom, and versatile anal sex roles in same-sex male relationships: Implications for relationship and sexual satisfaction. *Archives of Sexual Behavior, 48*(4), 1217–1225. https://doi.org/10.1007/s10508-018-1240-5

Moskowitz, D. A., Rieger, G., & Roloff, M. E. (2008). Tops, bottoms and versatiles. *Sexual and Relationship Therapy, 23*(3), 191–202. https://doi.org/10.1080/14681990802027259

Murphy, R. D., Gorbach, P. M., Weiss, R. E., Hucks-Ortiz, C., & Shoptaw, S. J. (2012). Seroadaptation in a sample of very poor Los Angeles area men who have sex with men. *AIDS and Behavior, 17*(5), 1862–1872. https://doi.org/10.1007/s10461-012-0213-2

Ober, A. J., Dangerfield, D. T., II, Shoptaw, S., Ryan, G., Stucky, B., & Friedman, S. R. (2018). Using a "Positive Deviance" framework to discover adaptive risk reduction behaviors among high-risk HIV negative Black men who have sex with men. *AIDS and Behavior, 22*(5), 1699–1712. https://doi.org/10.1007/s10461-017-1790-x

O'Cleirigh, C., Safren, S. A., & Mayer, K. H. (2012). The pervasive effects of childhood sexual abuse: Challenges for improving HIV prevention and treatment interventions. *Journal of Acquired Immune Deficiency Syndromes (1999), 59*(4), 331–334. https://doi.org/10.1097/QAI.0b013e31824aed80

Pachankis, J. E., Buttenwieser, I. G., Bernstein, L. B., & Bayles, D. O. (2013). A longitudinal, mixed methods study of sexual position identity, behavior, and fantasies among young sexual minority men. *Archives of Sexual Behavior, 42*(7), 1241–1253. https://doi.org/10.1007/s10508-013-0090-4

Parsons, J. T., Severino, J., Nanin, J., Punzalan, J. C., von Sternberg, K., Missildine, W., & Frost, D. (2006). Positive, negative, unknown: Assumptions of HIV status among HIV-positive men who have sex with men. *AIDS Education and Prevention: Official Publication of the International Society for AIDS Education, 18*(2), 139–149. https://doi.org/10.1521/aeap.2006.18.2.139

Phillips, G., Magnus, M., Kuo, I., Rawls, A., Peterson, J., Montanez, L., West-Ojo, T., Jia, Y., Opoku, J., & Greenberg, A. E. (2014). Childhood sexual abuse and HIV-related risks among men who have sex with men in Washington, DC. *Archives of Sexual Behavior, 43*(4), 771–778. https://doi.org/10.1007/s10508-014-0267-5

Relf, M. V. (2001). Childhood sexual abuse in men who have sex with men: The current state of the science. *Journal of the Association of Nurses in AIDS Care, 12*(5), 20–29. https://doi.org/10.1016/S1055-3290(06)60260-4

Shaw, L., Wang, L., Cui, Z., Rich, A. J., Armstrong, H. L., Lachowsky, N. J., Sereda, P., Card, K. G., Olarewaju, G., Moore, D., Hogg, R., & Roth, E. A. (2019). Longitudinal event-level analysis of gay and bisexual men's anal sex versatility: Behavior, roles, and substance use. *The Journal of Sex Research, 1–11*. https://doi.org/10.1080/00224499.2019.1652238

Simon, W., & Gagnon, J. H. (1984). Sexual scripts. *Society, 22*(1), 53–60. https://doi.org/10.1007/BF02701260

Sullivan, P. S., Driggers, R., Stekler, J. D., Siegler, A., Goldenberg, T., McDougal, S. J., Caucutt, J., Jones, J., & Stephenson, R. (2017). Usability and acceptability of a mobile comprehensive HIV prevention app for men who have sex with men: A pilot study. *JMIR mHealth and uHealth, 5*(3), e7199. https://doi.org/10.2196/mhealth.7199

Truong, N., Perez-Brumer, A., Burton, M., Gipson, J., & Hickson, D. (2016). What is in a label? Multiple meanings of 'MSM' among same-gender-loving Black men in Mississippi. *Global Public Health, 11*(7–8), 937–952. https://doi.org/10.1080/17441692.2016.1142593

Unemo, M., & Nicholas, R. A. (2012). Emergence of multidrug-resistant, extensively drug-resistant and untreatable gonorrhea. *Future Microbiology, 7*(12), 1401–1422. https://doi.org/10.2217/fmb.12.117

Vallabhaneni, S., Li, X., Vittinghoff, E., Donnell, D., Pilcher, C. D., & Buchbinder, S. P. (2012). Seroadaptive practices: Association with HIV acquisition among HIV-negative men who have sex with men. *PLoS ONE, 7*(10), e45718. https://doi.org/10.1371/journal.pone.0045718

Van de Ven, P., Kippax, S., Crawford, J., Rawstorne, P., Prestage, G., Grulich, A., & Murphy, D. (2002). In a minority of gay men, sexual risk practice indicates strategic positioning for perceived risk reduction rather than unbridled sex. *AIDS Care, 14*(4), 471–480. https://doi.org/10.1080/09540120208629666

van Druten, H., van Griensven, F., & Hendriks, J. (1992). Homosexual role separation: Implications for analyzing and modeling the spread of HIV. *The Journal of Sex Research, 29*(4), 477–499. https://doi.org/10.1080/00224499209551663

Vittinghoff, E., Douglas, J., Judson, F., McKirnan, D., MacQueen, K., & Buchbinder, S. P. (1999). Per-contact risk of human immunodeficiency virus transmission between male sexual partners. *American Journal of Epidemiology, 150*(3), 306–311.

Vosburgh, H. W., Mansergh, G., Sullivan, P. S., & Purcell, D. W. (2012). A review of the literature on event-level substance use and sexual risk behavior among men who have sex with men. *AIDS and Behavior, 16*(6), 1394–1410. https://doi.org/10.1007/s10461-011-0131-8

Wade, R. M., & Nguyễn, D. M. (2024). Does subjective racial attraction vary by sexual position? An analysis of young sexual minority Black men. *Sexuality & Culture, 28*(4), 1775–1791. https://doi.org/10.1007/s12119-024-10205-3

Wegesin, D. J., & Meyer-Bahlburg, H. F. L. (2000). Top/bottom self-label, anal sex practices, HIV risk and gender role identity in gay men in New York City. *Journal of Psychology & Human Sexuality, 12*(3), 43–62. https://doi.org/10.1300/J056v12n03_03

Wei, C., & Raymond, H. F. (2010). Preference for and maintenance of anal sex roles among men who have sex with wen: Sociodemographic and behavioral correlates. *Archives of Sexual Behavior, 40*(4), 829–834. https://doi.org/10.1007/s10508-010-9623-2

Wei, C., Raymond, H. F., Guadamuz, T. E., Stall, R., Colfax, G. N., Snowden, J. M., & McFarland, W. (2010). Racial/Ethnic differences in seroadaptive and serodisclosure behaviors among men who have sex with men. *AIDS and Behavior, 15*(1), 22–29. https://doi.org/10.1007/s10461-010-9683-2

Wheeler, D. P., Lauby, J. L., Liu, K., Van Sluytman, L. G., & Murrill, C. (2008). A Comparative analysis of sexual risk characteristics of Black men who have sex with men or with men and women. *Archives of Sexual Behavior, 37*(5), 697–707. https://doi.org/10.1007/s10508-008-9372-7

Wilken, J. A., Ried, C., Rickett, P., Arno, J. N., Mendez, Y., Harrison, R. J., Wohlfeiler, D., Bauer, H. M., Joyce, M. P., Switzer, W. M., Heneine, W., Shankar, A., & Mark, K. E. (2016). Occupational HIV transmission among male adult film performers—Multiple states, 2014. *MMWR. Morbidity and Mortality Weekly Report, 65*(5), 110–114. https://doi.org/10.15585/mmwr.mm6505a3

Wilson, P. A., Valera, P., Ventuneac, A., Balan, I., Rowe, M., & Carballo-Diéguez, A. (2009). Race-based sexual stereotyping and sexual partnering among men who use the internet to identify other men for bareback sex. *The Journal of Sex Research, 46*(5), 399–413. https://doi.org/10.1080/00224490902846479

Winder, T. J. A. (2023). The discursive work of "Bottom-Shaming": Sexual positioning discourse in the construction of black masculinity. *Gender & Society, 37*(5), 774–799. https://doi.org/10.1177/08912432231186999

Wingood, G. M., & DiClemente, R. J. (2000). Application of the theory of gender and power to examine HIV-related exposures, risk factors, and effective interventions for women. *Health Education & Behavior, 27*(5), 539–565. https://doi.org/10.1177/109019810002700502

Zablotska, I. B., Imrie, J., Prestage, G., Crawford, J., Rawstorne, P., Grulich, A., Jin, F., & Kippax, S. (2009). Gay men's current practice of HIV seroconcordant unprotected anal intercourse: Serosorting or seroguessing? *AIDS Care, 21*(4), 501–510. https://doi.org/10.1080/09540120802270292

Chapter 2
Theorizing Sexual Health Vulnerability, Redefining Risk, and Identifying Research Question(s)

Chapter Objectives

1. Critically examine traditional definitions and measures of HIV/STI risk for Black sexual minority men (SMM).
2. Review existing theories and concepts regarding sexual health vulnerability among Black SMM.
3. Formulate and prioritize research questions to address knowledge gaps

Disease Risk versus Disease Vulnerability

Disease risk refers to the likelihood or probability that an individual (or population) will develop a particular health condition (e.g., HIV or other STIs) within a specified period of time (Rothman et al., 2008). For example, modeling data suggested that U.S. Black SMM have an estimated 50% and lifetime *risk* of HIV acquisition if treatment and prevention activities do not substantially improve (Hess et al., 2017). Assessing and understanding risk is essential for disease prevention, screening, and detection to reduce morbidity and mortality. By studying the patterns of disease incidence and identifying risk factors that are associated with acquisition, prevention scientists can design targeted interventions to improve population health outcomes and reduce sexual health disparities. While disease risk focuses on the probability of disease based on individual behaviors or environmental exposures, disease *vulnerability* examines broader social, cultural, and structural factors that shape individuals' susceptibility or ability to prevent disease (Adger, 2006). Factors of vulnerability can include socio-economic status, racism, stigma, lack of healthcare access, and other social determinants of health (Beyrer et al., 2012; Millett et al., 2012). Structural factors such as criminalizing behaviors (e.g., same-sex

D. T. Dangerfield II, *Prevention Science & Targeted Methods for HIV/STI Research with Black Sexual Minority Men*,
https://doi.org/10.1007/978-3-031-85130-8_2

sexuality) and lack of comprehensive sex education also contribute to disease vulnerability (Beyrer et al., 2012). Vulnerable populations can refer to marginalized groups such as sex workers, transgender individuals, people who inject drugs, and racial and sexual minorities, all of whom face disproportionate barriers to accessing prevention, screening, and treatment services (Beyrer et al., 2013; Meyer, 2007; Rhodes, 2002; Risher et al., 2015). Sexual health prevention science can be more comprehensive, equitable, and impactful by addressing both disease risk and vulnerability, especially for marginalized communities. This chapter provides some information regarding the role of relevant frameworks in the study of HIV/STI risk and vulnerability among Black SMM.

Reconceptualizing Sexual "Risk" Among Black Sexual Minority Men

Although disease risk and vulnerability are related concepts, they should not be used interchangeably in sexual health research with Black SMM. The reason for this is that risk primarily quantifies the probability of disease occurrence based on specific behaviors or exposures, while vulnerability encompasses a broader range of factors—including social, economic, and structural determinants—that predispose individuals to adverse health outcomes. Using these terms interchangeably can obscure the nuanced interplay of cultural dynamics, social inequalities, and access barriers that uniquely marginalize Black SMM, leading to oversimplified analyses and limited interventions. The ways in which prevention scientists conceptualize "risk" among Black SMM require further examination and consideration because the conventional measures of risk such as condomless sex have not explained racial/ethnic differences in HIV/STI incidence for this group (Maulsby et al., 2013; Millett et al., 2007, 2012; Sullivan et al., 2014). Instead, the research on the factors that constitute risk among Black SMM has produced two distinct streams of findings. On one hand, systematic reviews and meta-analyses have underscored that Black SMM demonstrate protective sexual health behaviors. For more than a decade, data have consistently showed that Black SMM use condoms more, have fewer sex partners, and use drugs less frequently before or during sex than others (Maulsby et al., 2013; Millett et al., 2007, 2012; Sullivan et al., 2014). On the other hand, additional studies show that other socioecological factors such as age, behavioral health, racism, stigma, and healthcare inaccess increase STI/HIV vulnerability for Black SMM (Ericksen & Trocki, 1992; Leichliter et al., 2020; Sullivan et al., 2014). Collectively, the literature suggests that contextual factors create a conundrum regarding why sexual health disparities persist for this community. Therefore, it is imperative to move beyond simplistic behavioral metrics to understand the nuanced and intersecting socioecological factors that contribute to sexual health disparities among Black SMM. By integrating a broader spectrum of influences, such as nuanced cultural dynamics regarding sexuality (See Chap. 1), socio-economic conditions, and the psychosocial factors, prevention scientists can better identify and address the root causes of these disparities. There is also a need for innovative methodologies and interventions targeting the unique experiences of Black SMM. Comprehensive methodological approaches must not only acknowledge the protective behaviors among Black SMM but also highlight the structural and social determinants that undermine prevention activities.

In light of the decades of research highlighting inequities in sexual health outcomes among SMM, the advances in STI/HIV treatment and prevention have also changed the contemporary sexual risk environment (Rhodes, 2002) and sexual health vulnerabilities for the general population. For example, HIV treatment has progressed from a toxic multi-pill regimen to a once daily safe dose that substantially reduces HIV in the blood; people living with HIV who have an undetectable viral load do not transmit the virus to their partners (Eisinger et al., 2019). Additionally, the U.S. Food and Drug Administration (FDA) approved the HIV treatment drug called Truvada for pre-exposure prophylaxis (PrEP) in 2012 to reduce acquisition risk. In 2019, the FDA also approved Descovy, a smaller HIV treatment pill for PrEP that demonstrated fewer side effects (Mayer et al., 2020). Recently, the FDA approved long-acting injectable versions of both PrEP and HIV treatment that are safe, effective, and improve medication adherence (Kirby, 2020; US FDA, 2021). A growing literature also shows that use of doxycycline within 72 of sexual activity substantially reduces risk for gonorrhea, chlamydia, and syphilis (Bolan et al., 2015; Grant et al., 2020). These effective biomedical prevention options have the contemporary sexual "riskcape" for this population (Hickson et al., 2015) by reducing transmission risks, improving life expectancy and quality of life, and reducing fear and stigma. However, Black SMM remain disproportionately more vulnerable to HIV and STIs than the general population and solutions to reduce disparities remain elusive. A pressing public health research question remains: "*What mutable factors can account for the increased and differential HIV/STI vulnerability among Black gay and bisexual men?*"

Key Theoretical Frameworks for Sexual Health Prevention Science and Intervention Design

Studies (including interventions) that are theoretically guided are crucial for prevention science, health promotion, health education, and public health programming. Theory is crucial to identifying the necessary points for research and intervention strategies because they help scientists and public health practitioners understand why people behave the way they do or have particular experiences that increase their disease vulnerability. Theoretically guided approaches can achieve population-level impact and inform sustainable prevention efforts over time. In prevention science, solutions can be designed based upon theories from several disciplines, including psychology, sociology, and communication. The role of classic theoretical frameworks is becoming increasingly overlooked in the recent STI/HIV prevention science literature as contemporary interventions emphasize the use of implementation science frameworks to improve uptake of biomedical interventions (Charest et al., 2021; Golub & Myers, 2019; Sullivan et al., 2019). Moreover, studies are moving away from behavior change models to focus more on "social and structural" factors that impact health outcomes Black SMM (Arrington-Sanders et al., 2020; Bowleg et al., 2022; Brewer et al., 2019; Hotton et al., 2020) given the data highlighting inequities in risk behaviors and outcomes. However, some contemporary implementation science approaches lack key theoretical underpinnings that identify the behavior change mechanisms of interventions success for individuals and communities. Additionally, individual-level factors and the antecedents of behavior are often easier to identify, target, and modify through public health interventions, whereas structural factors like "racism" and "stigma" are more entrenched, complex, and challenging to address within a short timeframe. Therefore, the following section will highlight how classic theories can be used to effectively and systematically support Black SMM.

Health Behavior Theory: The Health Belief Model

Not everyone gets vaccinated or takes a prescribed prophylactic medication (e.g., PrEP for HIV prevention). The differences in why some people engage in health behaviors or not can be rooted in a cognitive decision-making process in which a person weighs the pros and cons of prevention behaviors. Identifying this process has led to theories such as the Health Belief Model (HBM) to account for differences in prevention behaviors using the cognitive construct of risk perceptions (Ferrer & Klein, 2015; Maiman & Becker, 1974). According to the HBM, the health behavior decision making involves perceived susceptibility (i.e., the likelihood of getting a disease), perceived severity (i.e., the seriousness of contracting an illness), benefits of actions to reduce STI threats (how effective an action will be to reduce susceptibility), and perceived barriers (impediments that may reduce the efficacy of action such as psychological or economic costs) (Rosenstock, 1974a). Another HBM construct involves cues to action, which are events that affect risk perceptions and trigger the decision-making process (Maiman & Becker, 1974; Rosenstock, 1974a; Rosenstock et al., 1994). Cues to action can be a placard in a subway station with a prevention message, a friend becoming ill, or a reminder from a clinic to get tested (Rosenstock, 1974a). Other crucial risk factors that may influence health beliefs include self-efficacy and locus of control (Elopre et al., 2021; Rosenstock et al., 1994). The HBM posits that a person deliberates over health behaviors because they want something of value (i.e., to avoid illness) and they consider the various actions to obtain the outcome. The HBM helped prevention scientists understand how women needing mammograms weighed the cost (e.g., traveling, missing work, co-pays) against whether they believed they were at risk for breast cancer (Darvishpour et al., 2018). The HBM has also been used to effectively address sunscreen use, medication adherence, dietary control, condom use, and other prevention behaviors in general populations (Hall, 2012; Janz & Becker, 1984; Rosenstock et al., 1994). Decades of research show that behaviors can be changed by using relevant frameworks, valid measures, and interventions that adequately address the antecedents of change.

Generating Research Questions Based Upon the Health Belief Model

Missing from the two streams of thought regarding HIV vulnerability for Black SMM is a focus on the cognitive elements of risk, the deliberative processes that people engage as they consider different sexual health behaviors. This is highly significant and requires attention because some HIV-negative Black SMM believe that they are not vulnerable to STIs because they have not acquired HIV and because they have relatively "lower" numbers of partners than their past and their peers (Dangerfield II et al., 2022a; Ober et al., 2018). Some Black SMM perceive STIs as less severe than HIV given the advances in HIV treatment and the proliferation of the global HIV stigma reduction campaign "U=U" that emphasizes the science that individuals with an undetectable viral load cannot transmit the virus (Boom et al., 2013; Daar & Corado, 2016; Dangerfield II et al., 2022a). Data also show that some Black SMM trust their subjective estimates regarding their sexual partners' STI/HIV status (Dangerfield II et al., 2022a; Ober et al., 2018). These studies reinforce that Black SMM cognitively place emphasis contextual factors that could contribute to observed health inequities in the U.S. but this remains unaddressed in the prevention science literature. The HBM could be a useful value-expectancy framework to design studies that target key cognitive precursors of decision making for Black SMM given the optional nature of contemporary prevention strategies such as PrEP.

Given their integral role in the deliberation process, health beliefs are a promising target for STI prevention research among Black SMM (Dangerfield II & Anderson, 2024). Some may participate in a cognitive value-expectancy process regarding STI prevention behaviors. The value "*I want to have sex with this person but I don't want syphilis*" can be weighed against the expectancy "*I don't know their sexual history, what could potentially happen?*" The costs of an STI could also outweigh the benefits of sexual risk taking and promulgate an action to engage in protective behavior (i.e., condom use, abstinence, or doxycycline post-exposure prophylaxis [doxy-PEP]). According to the HBM, perceived disease severity is required for individuals to engage in prevention behaviors (e.g., condom use and post exposure prophylaxis [i.e., doxy-PEP]) (Alizade et al., 2021; Rosenstock et al., 1994). However, the cognitive elements of decision-making and how Black SMM perceive their STI "risk" remains understudied. Although sexual health prevention science is moving away from behavior change models to focus on social and structural factors, the HBM suggests that factors such as socioeconomic status can be overcome with appropriate use of the model (Rosenstock, 1974a, b). Moreover, changing structural drivers of health disparities such as racism and discrimination may be beyond the scope of individual research protocols. Therefore, the HBM is a crucial framework in health promotion and disease prevention for racial and sexual minority men that cannot be overlooked.

Example Research Guided by the Health Belief Model

Between 2021 and 2023, I pilot tested a multicomponent intervention called POSSIBLE to improve perceived HIV risk and PrEP initiation among Black SMM in Baltimore, MD (Dangerfield II et al., 2024). POSSILBLE was a virtual, two-session, single-group feasibility intervention designed to leverage a peer change agent (PCA) and a mobile smartphone app to cue individuals to action by recording and reviewing the sexual histories in an app-based diary with the PCA. POSSIBLE involved two study visits conducted 1 month a part. Baseline study visits involved a 20-minute motivational interview-based script with a PrEP-using PCA to discuss relative HIV risk behaviors, perceived HIV risk, health information, and PrEP with Black SMM. The goals of the PCA were to anticipate and respond to multilevel barriers and to introduce PrEP as a beneficial option that supports their health holistically. Study visits followed a motivational interview-techniques to provide health information, incorporate PrEP within participant goals, and encourage PrEP use regardless of their behaviors (Dangerfield II et al., 2022a, 2023; Dangerfield II, 2023). Participants were asked HIV vulnerability questions such as "*What do you think about your HIV risk given that estimates suggest that 50% of Black SMM will acquire it*?" to identify HIV prevention intentions. Results showed a statistically significant increase in perceived HIV risk after the first session before they downloaded the app. Additionally, 64% were willing to be referred to PrEP services after the baseline session, 45% of whom had a confirmed PrEP appointment. These data are highly promising because they suggest that health beliefs including risk perceptions are a promising target for intervention that is quickly mutable, hopefully leading to significant community impact.

Intersectionality for the Prevention Science Discipline

Intersectionality is a crucial framework for HIV prevention research, particularly when examining the unique challenges faced by Black SMM. Originally rooted in the legal discipline, intersectionality was developed by scholar Kimberlé Crenshaw to highlight how Black women's experiences were overlooked in both feminist and antiracist movements (Crenshaw, 1991). Crenshaw argued that legal frameworks often failed to address the compounded discrimination faced by individuals at the intersections of multiple marginalized identities. This perspective has since expanded into public health and social sciences, offering a powerful lens to examine how overlapping social identities—such as race, gender, sexual orientation, and socioeconomic status—shape experiences and vulnerabilities (Bowleg, 2013, 2021; Bowleg et al., 2022). Black SMM often navigate structural inequalities including racism, homophobia, and economic disparities, which compound their vulnerability and limit their access to healthcare and prevention resources. Intersectionality recognizes the interconnected and overlapping social identities—such as race, gender, sexual orientation, and socioeconomic status—that shape individuals' experiences and HIV/STI vulnerability. It can guide the design of studies and interventions that address the root causes of vulnerability, including racism and discrimination, while also recognizing the resilience and agency within the community. This holistic perspective fosters more equitable and effective prevention efforts, ensuring that the complexities of identity and systemic oppression are central to reducing HIV disparities in this community.

The Socioecological Model (SEM)

As mentioned at the beginning of the chapter, the health outcomes of Black SMM are not exclusively explained by behavioral differences. Instead, social and structural factors in society affect health disparities and inequalities in the community. Social theories such as the Socio-Ecological Model (SEM, Bronfenbrenner, 1979) can help explain how the communities and contexts influence the health outcomes of Black SMM. The SEM examines the interplay between social determinants of health on multiple levels: the individual, relationship, community, and societal (Bronfenbrenner, 1979; Centers for Disease Control and Prevention, 2019). The individual level focuses on biological, demographic, and personal factors such as age, sex, education, and income. The interpersonal level examines close relationships including peers, partners, and family members who can influence behavior. The community level explores settings such as the built environment, neighborhoods, and healthcare organizations where people live, work, or socialize. The societal level focuses on broad factors such as cultural norms regarding sexual and gender minorities, healthcare policies, and other social policies that help maintain economic or social inequalities between social groups. In addition to clarifying multiple social and ecological factors of influence, the SEM also suggests that these levels overlap; factors at one level influence factors at another level. Therefore, it would be necessary to research and act across multiple levels (at least 2) simultaneously to improve the health of Black SMM (Centers for Disease Control and Prevention, 2019; Pinto et al., 2018). This multifaceted approach suggests that interventions targeting only individual behaviors may not fully address the broader systemic issues contributing to health disparities. By integrating efforts across all levels of the SEM, public health strategies can more effectively mitigate the complex social and structural determinants that disproportionately affect Black SMM.

Generating Research Questions Based Upon the Socioecological Model and Intersectionality

Studies consistently show that Black SMM throughout the U.S. anticipate and experience racism and intersectional (i.e., sexuality and HIV) stigma on individual, relationship, community, and structural socio-ecological levels (Arnold et al., 2014; Bowleg et al., 2022; Quinn et al., 2018). For example, Black SMM who are living with HIV also experience rejection and social isolation from peers due HIV stigma that labels them as "dirty" or "reckless" (Arscott et al., 2019; Koester et al., 2018; Winder & Lea, 2019). Romantic/sexual partners demonstrate racism and intersectional stigma when they reject Black SMM living with HIV as "unsafer" than non-Black partners (Winder & Lea, 2019). In healthcare settings, clinicians are more likely to use stigmatizing language, ignore treatment requests, and withhold novel treatments from Black patients than white patients (Beach et al., 2011; Cooper et al., 2012; Johnson et al., 2004; Shen et al., 2018). Racism and intersectional stigma increase medical mistrust and decrease willingness to accept clinicians' treatment recommendations (Dale et al., 2016; Hammond et al., 2010; Quinn et al., 2018). Black SMM also have lower access to resourceful HIV care facilities than white patients (Hoffman et al., 2016; Maina et al., 2018; Shen et al., 2018; Sullivan et al., 2021). Moreover, policies such as Medicaid non-expansion, HIV criminalization laws, and clinic billing practices create structural barriers for low-resourced men living with HIV (Bowleg et al., 2022). The rejection, discrimination, and stigma from family, peers, potential partners, and clinicians due to race, sexuality, and HIV status reduce their treatment adherence because Black SMM living with HIV become depressed and hopeless and use drugs and alcohol to cope (Ferlatte et al., 2017; Quinn et al., 2016; Quinn & Voisin, 2020; Voisin et al., 2017). Some simply stop taking their medication to avoid the HIV stigma associated with being on treatment (Dangerfield II et al., 2020). Uptake of effective contemporary medications such as the new, long-acting Cabenuva injectable antiretroviral medication will likely be slow for Black SMM living with HIV unless these barriers are addressed. Therefore, it is crucial to design and implement interventions that not only address individual-level behaviors but also actively dismantle the pervasive racism and intersectional stigma embedded within social, relational, community, and structural contexts. Without comprehensive strategies that target these broader determinants of health, Black SMM living with HIV will continue to face significant obstacles to achieving optimal health outcomes. Prioritizing equity in healthcare access, reducing stigma, and fostering supportive environments at all levels of society are essential steps toward ensuring that advancements in HIV treatment, like the Cabenuva injectable, are accessible and beneficial to all individuals, regardless of race or socioeconomic status.

Social science frameworks such Intersectionality as Critical Race Theory (CRT) suggest that some communities have marginalized identities (e.g., Black race, gay identification, and HIV status) that create negative socio-ecological experiences everywhere even if they do not know it (Airhihenbuwa & Ford, 2018; Bowleg, 2013; Ford & Airhihenbuwa, 2010). We can combine the tenets of the Socioecological Model, Intersectionality, and CRT into a Conceptual Model (Fig. 2.1) that focuses on the Individual (i.e., intrapersonal and behavioral), Relationship (i.e., social support, patient-clinician communication), and Community (i.e., neighborhood and clinic factors) socioecological levels because they are the most feasible for researchers to impact in intervention designs and more quickly mutable as needed. CRT suggests that racism is the greatest barrier for Black SMM who are living with HIV (Airhihenbuwa & Ford, 2018; Ford & Airhihenbuwa, 2010); stigma should be added

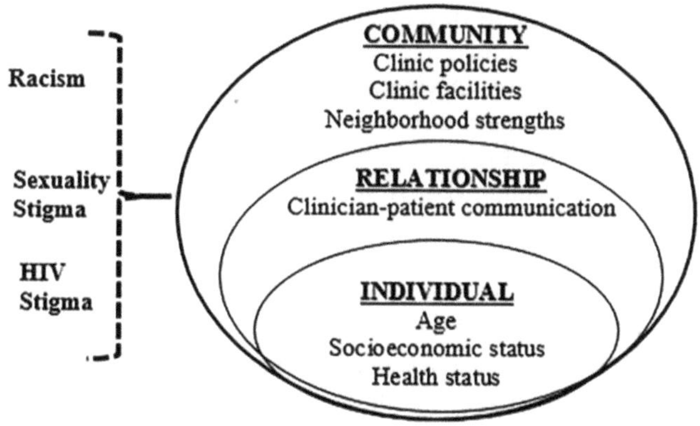

Fig. 2.1 Conceptual model of a combined framework incorporating SEM, Intersectionality, and CRT

as a multilevel barrier conceptually because the intersectional identities of race, sexuality, and HIV status expose Black SMM to racism and stigma in tandem and cannot be isolated, especially for those who are living with HIV (Bowleg, 2013; Quinn et al., 2019). Traditional understandings of the social determinants of sexual health for should be updated when studying Black SMM because racism and intersectional stigma are salient for this group and affect all levels of their social ecology (Bowleg, 2013; Bowleg et al., 2022; Randolph et al., 2020). Prevention scientists must use frameworks that can better capture the complex interplay of factors that shape the health experiences of Black SMM. This approach not only acknowledges the deep-rooted impact of racism and stigma but also provides a framework for designing interventions that address these barriers at multiple socioecological levels, ultimately leading to more equitable and effective health outcomes for Black SMM.

Positive Deviance: A Strengths-Based Framework

An emerging approach in public health emphasizes the importance of recognizing and building upon the inherent strengths of individuals and communities (Ezell et al., 2023; Liboro et al., 2021; Poteat & Logie, 2022). Strengths-based research frameworks focus on identifying and leveraging individuals' and communities' existing assets and resources to promote positive outcomes and address challenges. These frameworks emphasize a shift away from deficit-based approaches that focus solely on identifying problems toward approaches that emphasize empowerment and capacity building. For example, Positive Deviance examines uncommon behaviors among those with better outcomes than their peers despite having comparable risks for adverse outcomes (Friedman et al., 2008; Marsh et al., 2004; Ober et al.,

2018). Theoretically, "positive deviants" have existing individual-level strengths that could help them overcome barriers in uncommon or unconscious ways. Approaches guided by Positive Deviance identify individuals with better outcomes than their peers, interview them to discover adaptive and presumably uncommon behaviors, and confirm that the behaviors are unusual but effective. This information is then used for community-driven interventions (von Hippel, 2018). This method not only highlights successful practices within the community but also fosters a sense of ownership and empowerment among participants, as the solutions are derived from within the community itself rather than being imposed externally. By focusing on these effective, yet often overlooked behaviors, Positive Deviance approaches can inspire broader adoption of these practices, leading to sustainable and culturally relevant improvements in health and well-being across the community. These interventions, rooted in the real-life experiences of those who have successfully navigated challenges, are more likely to resonate with others facing similar obstacles and result in meaningful, long-term change.

Example Positive Deviance Study in Prevention Research with Black SMM

I led an NINR-sponsored study exploring explicit strategies that virally suppressed Black SMM who were living with HIV used to maintain treatment adherence in Baltimore, MD and Los Angeles, CA (Dangerfield II et al., 2022b). The premise of the study was based on the understanding that despite the significant challenges of retention in care, achieving viral suppression, and navigating systemic disparities, some Black SMM who were living with HIV successfully managed their care. The study aimed to explore the strategies, behaviors, and support systems that enabled their success. The goal was to identify actionable insights and strengths-based approaches that could inform interventions for Black SMM who had trouble being retained in care or adhering to treatment. Study domains focused on uncovering explicit behaviors and strategies for overcoming socioecological barriers including substance use, poor mental health, and healthcare access. In-depth interviews revealed that they used intentional, age group-specific treatment adherence strategies such as using technology (among men age ≤ 35) and taking HIV medications with other daily pills (among men age > 35). Men across age groups also described a desire to live for themselves or loved ones became a symbiotic goal that helped them sustain their ART adherence. Of note, most men in that study described suicide ideation upon receiving their HIV diagnosis but described how social support, spirituality, and personal goals in life improved their will to live and subsequently adhere to treatment. Hypothetically, these could be components in an intervention to improve HIV care outcomes for this community.

I also conducted ethnographic go-along interviews to identify supportive clinical factors for virally suppressed Black SMM LWH in Baltimore, MD (Dangerfield II et al., 2021). The direct observations of HIV care visits during go-alongs contradicted previous in-depth interview data that suggested participants had "good" clinical experiences because I <u>saw</u> that Black SMM LWH navigated dissatisfying experiences by being dishonest to maintain healthcare access. For example, participants travelled far distances on public transportation, expressed discomfort during long wait times, and navigated dissatisfying treatment from clinicians to obtain their prescriptions and access clinic resources (Dangerfield II et al., 2021). They also anticipated unsatisfactory, stigmatizing communication in their clinical experiences and used preemptive conversations to mitigate their discomfort so that their conversation continued toward the goal of the clinic visit (i.e., obtaining their prescription). I did not find explicit derogatory language in their neighborhood or clinical experiences as studies of racialized experiences suggest. Instead, I found that participants perceived questions, pauses, or abruptly ending the visit as unsatisfactory, stigmatizing, or racist. These findings highlight the complexity of clinical interactions for Black SMM living with HIV, revealing that what might appear as "good" clinical experiences on the surface might, in reality, involve significant efforts by patients to navigate and mitigate discomfort and stigma. The implications of this research through the lens of Positive Deviance suggest that identifying and understanding the adaptive strategies (strengths) used by these patients could inform more effective and culturally sensitive interventions in clinical and community settings. Healthcare systems can be better equipped to reduce the need for such navigation and create environments that are genuinely supportive, reducing the burden on patients to adapt to less-than-ideal conditions and ultimately improving their overall healthcare experience and outcomes. Prevention scientists can also leverage the strategies that individuals use to navigate barriers in interventions to build similar skills among others in the community.

Generating Additional Research Questions Based Upon Positive Deviance

Classic approaches of Positive Deviance do not necessarily seek to change structural factors because positive deviants withstand socioecological barriers (Friedman et al., 2008; Marsh et al., 2004; von Hippel, 2018). Positive Deviance fits into the interest of leveraging resilience to support marginalized communities (Herrick et al., 2011, 2014; McNair et al., 2018). However, Positive Deviance advances other strengths-based frameworks (such as those based on resilience) because positive deviants may not have optimistic perspectives although they have "positive" outcomes. Given the ubiquitous nature of socio-ecological barriers in sexual health promotion, prevention science should study population exemplars who leverage strengths in conscious and unconscious ways in the midst of barriers. By generating research questions that focus on understanding the specific behaviors, strategies, and contextual factors that enable these positive deviants to achieve better outcomes, researchers can uncover actionable insights that may be applicable to the broader community. This approach can lead to the design of more effective interventions that not only address individual resilience and adaptability but also provide practical solutions that others can adopt, thereby enhancing overall health outcomes in marginalized communities facing similar socio-ecological challenges.

Life Course

Life Course is a social science and developmental psychology framework to examine how historical, social, and environmental contexts and individual behavior impact outcomes (Elder, 1996, 1998). Life Course posits that behaviors and outcomes result from the individual, the environment, and time and include key constructs of timing, trajectories, transitions, and critical periods (Elder, 1996, 1998). This theory provides important guidance for understanding disease vulnerability among Black SMM because it orients researchers to examine how historical context creates particular age-related outcomes at critical periods along the life course (Dangerfield II et al., 2017, 2018). Moreover, Life Course emphasizes the cumulative impact of life experiences, suggesting that early-life exposures to violence, discrimination, stigma, or supportive environments can have lasting effects on health outcomes in later life. By integrating Life Course into research on Black SMM, prevention scientists can better understand how intersecting identities and experiences across different historical and social contexts shape health disparities. This approach also allows for the identification of critical periods where interventions may be most effective, offering a more nuanced understanding of how to promote health equity across the lifespan for these populations.

The Case for Examining Health Beliefs and Disease Vulnerability Over the Life Course

Most of my studies have focused on life theoretical approaches because generational differences in exposure to risk, coupled with the changing messaging about HIV risk and same-sex relationships create unique sexual risk environments among different generations of Black SMM. For example, Baby Boomer and Generation X (born prior to the 1980s) came of age during the first generation of the HIV/AIDS epidemic and witnessed terminal consequences of infection, since most people came to medical attention in the later stages of disease when effective treatments were unavailable. Comparatively, Millennials, Generation Z, and Generation Alpha witnessed a different epidemic in which HIV became increasingly treatable and subsequently more preventable. Younger generations of sexual minority individuals are also developing during a time in which social and structural changes such as the legalization of same-sex marriage reflect a more tolerant social climate regarding same-sex relationships (Glick et al., 2015). Given these historical and generational differences, a growing literature suggests that young gay, bisexual, and other sexual minorities might be more likely to engage in risk behaviors due to HIV optimism or complacency coupled with increased ability to meet partners and develop relationships (Callander & Senn, 2013; Dangerfield II et al., 2017; Nelson et al., 2016). Studies reinforce that Black SMM place emphasis on these and other personal and contextual factors that could contribute to observed health inequities (Boom et al.,

2013; Dangerfield II et al., 2022a; Ober et al., 2018). For example, some Black SMM perceive STIs as less severe than HIV given the global public health campaign "U=U" (Boom et al., 2013; Daar & Corado, 2016; Dangerfield II et al., 2022a). The Prevention Access Campaign launched the "U=U" campaign that was promoted by the World Health Organization to reduce HIV stigma by emphasizing that individuals with an undetectable viral load are untransmittible to their partners (Eisinger et al., 2019; National Institute of Allergy and Infectious Diseases, 2019). Given these generational differences, young SMM might be more likely to engage in risk behaviors due to feelings of HIV not being as lethal as it was initially, coupled with their increased ability to meet partners and develop relationship (Callander & Senn, 2013; Dangerfield II et al., 2017; Hammack & Cohler, 2011; Nelson et al., 2016). Younger age is also associated with sexual risk taking (Koblin et al., 2013; Mansergh & Marks, 1998; Mustanski et al., 2011; Osmond et al., 2007). It seems appropriate and timely, then, that we explore the social and sexual lives of Black SMM with a life course theoretical lens to better understand how evolving perceptions of HIV, influenced by public health messages like "U=U," intersect with generational shifts in sexual behavior and partner-seeking practices. By applying this lens, we can gain deeper insights into how different age cohorts of Black SMM navigate the complexities of sexual health in a changing epidemiological and social landscape, and how these factors contribute to ongoing sexual health inequities within this population.

Possible Selves: A Transdisciplinary Framework

The concept of "possible selves" garnered attention from Markus and Nurius's work in the 1980s as part of social psychology's exploration of self-concept (Markus & Nurius, 1986). Possible selves refer to the future-oriented dimensions of self-perception, encompassing the ideas of who individuals hope to become, who they fear becoming, and who they expect to become. Possible selves help individuals envision the outcomes of their actions and align their behaviors with their desired identities. Possible selves bridge the gap between motivation and behavior by linking one's aspirations and fears to self-regulated, actionable steps. Rooted in the interplay between personal goals and social influences, this theory emphasizes how the sociocultural context shapes individuals' future self-images and motivates efforts toward achieving or avoiding certain outcomes. Possible selves has been used to help explain outcomes behavioral health and academic outcomes among adolescents (Oyserman et al., 2002, 2006) and provides a powerful framework for prevention science among Black SMM because it could help individuals articulate their hopes and fears for the future, which could be leveraged interventions to foster self-efficacy and improve health outcomes. For example, programs could provide images (or live examples of individuals) that encourage Black SMM to envision futures where they achieve optimal health, strong social connections, and financial stability, while identifying and mitigating fears related to HIV stigma, discrimination, or social isolation. This approach could guide prevention strategies that improve engagement in care, enhancing adherence to medication, and building supportive networks by fostering mental images of aspirational figures that might trigger self-regulating behaviors. By grounding interventions in the aspirational identities of Black SMM, possible selves ensures that prevention efforts are both empowering and culturally relevant, promoting sustained behavior change and improved health outcomes.

Conclusions

Both concepts of risk and vulnerability are important for understanding the complex dynamics of STI/HIV transmission and designing effective interventions that address not only individual behaviors but also the underlying social determinants of health. The distinction between disease risk and disease vulnerability among Black SMM is nuanced. The conventional use of disease risk in research often overlooks the complex socioecological factors influencing health outcomes for Black SMM. Prevention science must conceptualize sexual risk among Black SMM and consider how contextual factors play significant roles in HIV/STI disparities. To better understand how to improve health for the community, the use of relevant theoretical frameworks is crucial. Prevention science must draw upon frameworks from a range of disciplines to design more effective interventions for Black SMM.

Raised Questions

1. How do understandings of risk and vulnerability contribute to how prevention scientists approach sexual health promotion for Black SMM?
2. How significant are health beliefs and other cognitive factors in the midst of social and structural barriers for this group?
3. What role do classic behavior change theories have on contemporary sexual health promotion initiatives?

Chapter Summary

This chapter delves into the complexities of sexual health vulnerability and risk among Black SMM, aiming to redefine traditional concepts and develop more effective research questions. The chapter began by distinguishing between "disease risk," which quantifies the likelihood of disease based on specific behaviors, and "disease vulnerability," which considers broader social, cultural, and structural factors that influence susceptibility to disease. This distinction is crucial in understanding the persistent sexual health disparities faced by Black SMM. The chapter critiqued conventional measures of sexual health risk, such as condomless sex, for failing to fully explain the high incidence of HIV and STIs among Black SMM, despite their often protective sexual health behaviors. Instead, it emphasizes the need to incorporate health beliefs and other socio-ecological factors to fully understand and address these disparities. The chapter also explores the application of key theoretical frameworks, such as the Health Belief Model (HBM) and the Socio-Ecological Model (SEM) in addressing sexual health disparities. The HBM was highlighted for its utility in understanding the cognitive processes behind health behavior decisions, such as the use of PrEP for HIV prevention. The SEM was discussed as a tool for examining the multilevel influences on health, from individual behaviors to broader societal factors. Positive Deviance was also discussed as a strengths-based approached that focuses on identifying and replicating the strengths and adaptive behaviors of the community. The chapter concluded by encouraging the development of research questions that focus on understanding these complex interactions and designing interventions that are both effective and culturally relevant for Black SMM.

Key Points

1. **The distinction between disease risk and vulnerability**: The chapter highlights the difference between disease risk, which quantifies the likelihood of health conditions based on individual behaviors, and disease vulnerability, which considers broader social, cultural, and structural factors, such as racism and stigma, that contribute to susceptibility. This distinction is crucial for understanding health disparities among Black SMM.
2. **Reconceptualizing sexual risk for Black SMM**: Traditional measures of risk, like condomless sex, fail to fully explain high HIV/STI rates among Black SMM despite evidence of protective behaviors (e.g., higher condom use). The chapter argues for a shift in focus from individual behaviors to socio-ecological factors like stigma, discrimination, and healthcare access, which drive persistent health disparities.
3. **Importance of theoretically driven prevention science**: The chapter emphasizes the need for theoretically guided research in sexual health prevention. It advocates using frameworks such as the HBM and the SEM to inform interventions by understanding the cognitive and social determinants of health behaviors among Black SMM.
4. **Positive Deviance as a strengths-based approach**: Positive Deviance focuses on identifying and amplifying the strengths of individuals who achieve better outcomes despite similar risks. This approach can inspire community-driven interventions that leverage successful behaviors already present within marginalized groups, leading to more sustainable health improvements.

5. **Life Course and generational differences in sexual health risk and vulnerability**: Life Course is explored as a framework for understanding how historical, social, and environmental contexts influence health outcomes across different generations of Black SMM. The chapter discusses how generational differences in experiences with HIV and societal changes shape sexual behaviors and perceptions of risk, highlighting the need for age-specific interventions that account for these evolving dynamics.

References

Adger, W. N. (2006). Vulnerability. *Global Environmental Change, 16*(3), 268–281. https://doi.org/10.1016/j.gloenvcha.2006.02.006

Airhihenbuwa, C. O., & Ford, C. L. (2018). Editorial: Critical race theory—We are all others. *Ethnicity & Disease, 28*(Suppl 1), 219–222. https://doi.org/10.18865/ed.28.S1.219

Alizade, M., Farshbaf-Khalili, A., Malakouti, J., & Mirghafourvand, M. (2021). Predictors of preventive behaviors of AIDS/HIV based on health belief model constructs in women with high-risk sexual behaviors: A cross-sectional survey. *Journal of Education and Health Promotion, 10*, 446. https://doi.org/10.4103/jehp.jehp_1046_20

Arnold, E. A., Rebchook, G. M., & Kegeles, S. M. (2014). "Triply cursed": Racism, homophobia, and HIV-related stigma are barriers to regular HIV testing, treatment adherence, and disclosure among young Black gay men. *Culture, Health & Sexuality, 16*(6), 710–722. https://doi.org/10.1080/13691058.2014.905706

Arrington-Sanders, R., Hailey-Fair, K., Wirtz, A. L., Morgan, A., Brooks, D., Castillo, M., Trexler, C., Kwait, J., Dowshen, N., Galai, N., Beyrer, C., & Celentano, D. (2020). Role of structural marginalization, HIV stigma, and mistrust on HIV prevention and treatment among young Black Latinx men who have sex with men and transgender women: Perspectives from youth service providers. *AIDS Patient Care and STDs, 34*(1), 7–15. https://doi.org/10.1089/apc.2019.0165

Arscott, J., Humphreys, J., Merwin, E., & Relf, M. (2019). "That guy is gay and Black. That's a red flag." How HIV stigma and racism affect perception of risk among young Black men who have sex with men. *AIDS and Behavior*. https://doi.org/10.1007/s10461-019-02607-4

Beach, M. C., Saha, S., Korthuis, P. T., Sharp, V., Cohn, J., Wilson, I. B., Eggly, S., Cooper, L. A., Roter, D., Sankar, A., & Moore, R. (2011). Patient–provider communication differs for Black compared to white HIV-infected patients. *AIDS and Behavior, 15*(4), 805–811. https://doi.org/10.1007/s10461-009-9664-5

Beyrer, C., Baral, S. D., van Griensven, F., Goodreau, S. M., Chariyalertsak, S., Wirtz, A. L., & Brookmeyer, R. (2012). Global epidemiology of HIV infection in men who have sex with men. *The Lancet, 380*(9839), 367–377. https://doi.org/10.1016/S0140-6736(12)60821-6

Beyrer, C., Sullivan, P., Sanchez, J., Baral, S. D., Collins, C., Wirtz, A. L., Altman, D., Trapence, G., & Mayer, K. (2013). The increase in global HIV epidemics in MSM. *AIDS, 27*(17), 2665–2678. https://doi.org/10.1097/01.aids.0000432449.30239.fe

Bolan, R. K., Beymer, M. R., Weiss, R. E., Flynn, R. P., Leibowitz, A. A., & Klausner, J. D. (2015). Doxycycline prophylaxis to reduce incident syphilis among HIV-infected men who have sex with men who continue to engage in high risk sex: A randomized, controlled pilot study. *Sexually Transmitted Diseases, 42*(2), 98–103. https://doi.org/10.1097/OLQ.0000000000000216

Boom, W. V. D., Stolte, I. G., Witlox, R., Sandfort, T., Prins, M., & Davidovich, U. (2013). Undetectable viral load and the decision to engage in unprotected anal intercourse among HIV-positive MSM. *AIDS and Behavior, 17*(6), 2136–2142. https://doi.org/10.1007/s10461-013-0453-9

Bowleg, L. (2013). "Once you've blended the cake, you can't take the parts back to the main ingredients": Black gay and bisexual men's descriptions and experiences of intersectionality. *Sex Roles, 68*(11–12), 754–767. https://doi.org/10.1007/s11199-012-0152-4

Bowleg, L. (2021). Evolving intersectionality within public health: From analysis to action. *American Journal of Public Health, 111*(1), 88–90. https://doi.org/10.2105/AJPH.2020.306031

Bowleg, L., Malekzadeh, A. N., Mbaba, M., & Boone, C. A. (2022). Ending the HIV epidemic for all, not just some: Structural racism as a fundamental but overlooked social-structural determinant of the US HIV epidemic. *Current Opinion in HIV and AIDS, 17*(2), 40–45. https://doi.org/10.1097/COH.0000000000000724

Brewer, R., Daunis, C., Ebaady, S., Wilton, L., Chrestman, S., Mukherjee, S., Moore, M., Corrigan, R., & Schneider, J. (2019). Implementation of a socio-structural demonstration project to improve HIV outcomes among young Black men in the Deep South. *Journal of Racial and Ethnic Health Disparities, 6*(4), 775–789. https://doi.org/10.1007/s40615-019-00576-x

Bronfenbrenner, U. (1979). *The ecology of human development*. Harvard University Press.

Callander, D., & Senn, C. (2013). Examining the role of relationships, body image, closeness to HIV/AIDS, and HIV optimism in the sexual risks of young men who have sex with men. *Journal of HIV/Aids & Social Services, 12*(2), 205–223. https://doi.org/10.1080/15381501.2013.790869

Centers for Disease Control and Prevention. (2019, April 9). *Social Determinants of Health | CDC*. https://www.cdc.gov/socialdeterminants/index.htm

Charest, M., Sharma, M., Chris, A., Schnubb, A., Knox, D. C., Wilton, J., Shahin, R., Chan, A., Mishra, S., Grace, D., Bayoumi, A. M., Maxwell, J., Bogoch, I. I., & Tan, D. H. S. (2021). Decentralizing PrEP delivery: Implementation and dissemination strategies to increase PrEP uptake among MSM in Toronto, Canada. *PLOS ONE, 16*(3), e0248626. https://doi.org/10.1371/journal.pone.0248626

Cooper, L. A., Roter, D. L., Carson, K. A., Beach, M. C., Sabin, J. A., Greenwald, A. G., & Inui, T. S. (2012). The associations of clinicians' implicit attitudes about race with medical visit communication and patient ratings of interpersonal care. *American Journal of Public Health, 102*(5), 979–987. https://doi.org/10.2105/AJPH.2011.300558

Crenshaw, K. (1991). Mapping the margins: Intersectionality, identity politics, and violence against women of color. *Stanford Law Review, 43*(6), 1241–1299. https://doi.org/10.2307/1229039

Daar, E. S., & Corado, K. (2016). Condomless sex with virologically suppressed HIV-infected individuals: How safe is it? *JAMA, 316*(2), 149–151. https://doi.org/10.1001/jama.2016.5636

Dale, S. K., Bogart, L. M., Wagner, G. J., Galvan, F. H., & Klein, D. J. (2016). Medical mistrust is related to lower longitudinal medication adherence among African-American males with HIV. *Journal of Health Psychology, 21*(7), 1311–1321. https://doi.org/10.1177/1359105314551950

Dangerfield, D. T., II. (2023). A principal investigator as a PrEP-using peer change agent for HIV prevention among Black gay and bisexual men: An autoethnography. *International Journal of Environmental Research and Public Health, 20*(7), 7. https://doi.org/10.3390/ijerph20075309

Dangerfield, D. T., II, & Anderson, J. N. (2024). A scripted, PrEP-using peer change agent improves perceived risk for HIV and willingness to accept referrals quickly among Black sexual minority men: Preliminary findings from POSSIBLE. *AIDS and Behavior, 28*, 2156–2165. https://doi.org/10.1007/s10461-024-04313-2

Dangerfield, D. T., II, Smith, L. R., Anderson, J. N., Bruce, O. J., Farley, J., & Bluthenthal, R. (2017). Sexual positioning practices and sexual risk among Black gay and bisexual men: A life course perspective. *AIDS and Behavior, 22*(6), 1919–1931. https://doi.org/10.1007/s10461-017-1948-6

Dangerfield, D. T., II, Harawa, N. T., Fernandez, M. I., Hosek, S., Lauby, J., Joseph, H., Frank, H. G., & Bluthenthal, R. N. (2018). Age cohort differences in sexual behaviors among Black men who have sex with men and women. *The Journal of Sex Research, 55*(8), 1012–1021. https://doi.org/10.1080/00224499.2017.1423016

Dangerfield, D. T., II, Heidari, O., Cooper, J., Allen, S., & Lucas, G. M. (2020). Motivations for opioid and stimulant use among drug using Black sexual minority men: A life course perspective. *Drug and Alcohol Dependence, 215*, 108224. https://doi.org/10.1016/j.drugalcdep.2020.108224

Dangerfield, D. T., II, Ober, A. J., Anderson, J. N., Gorbach, P., & Bluthenthal, R. N. (2021). Observational "go-alongs" of follow-up HIV care visits of two virally suppressed Black sexual minority men. *Public Health Nursing., 39*, 153–160. https://doi.org/10.1111/phn.12960

Dangerfield, D. T., II, Anderson, J. N., Wylie, C., Arrington-Sanders, R., Bluthenthal, R. N., Beyrer, C., & Farley, J. E. (2022a). Refining a multicomponent intervention to increase perceived HIV risk and PrEP initiation: Focus group study among Black sexual minority men. *JMIR Formative Research, 6*(8), e34181. https://doi.org/10.2196/34181

Dangerfield, D. T., II, Ober, A. J., Li, M. J., Allen, S., & Bluthenthal, R. N. (2022b). HIV treatment adherence strategies among virally suppressed Black sexual minority men in Baltimore, Maryland, and Los Angeles, California: A theory-based qualitative study. *Journal of the Association of Nurses in AIDS Care, 33*(1), 54–62. https://doi.org/10.1097/JNC.0000000000000304

Dangerfield, D. T., II, Anderson, J. N., Wylie, C., Bluthenthal, R., Beyrer, C., & Farley, J. E. (2024). A multicomponent intervention (POSSIBLE) to improve perceived risk for HIV among Black sexual minority men: Feasibility and preliminary effectiveness pilot study. *JMIR Human Factors, 11*(1), e54739. https://doi.org/10.2196/54739

Dangerfield, D. T., Davis, G., Pandian, V., & Anderson, J. N. (2023). Using motivational interviewing to increase HIV PrEP initiation and adherence: A scoping review. *Prevention Science, 24*(7), 1365–1375. https://doi.org/10.1007/s11121-023-01554-w

Darvishpour, A., Vajari, S. M., & Noroozi, S. (2018). Can health belief model predict breast cancer screening behaviors? *Open Access Macedonian Journal of Medical Sciences, 6*(5), 949–953. https://doi.org/10.3889/oamjms.2018.183

Eisinger, R. W., Dieffenbach, C. W., & Fauci, A. S. (2019). HIV viral load and transmissibility of HIV infection: Undetectable equals untransmittable. *JAMA, 321*(5), 451–452. https://doi.org/10.1001/jama.2018.21167

Elder, G. H. (1998). The life course as developmental theory. *Child Development, 69*(1), 1–12. https://doi.org/10.2307/1132065

Elder, G. H., Jr. (1996). Human lives in changing societies: Life course and developmental insights. In R. B. Cairns, G. H. Elder Jr., & E. J. Costello (Eds.), *Developmental science* (pp. 31–62). Cambridge University Press.

Elopre, L., Ott, C., Lambert, C. C., Amico, K. R., Sullivan, P. S., Marrazzo, J., Mugavero, M. J., & Turan, J. M. (2021). Missed prevention opportunities: Why young, Black MSM with recent HIV diagnosis did not access HIV pre-exposure prophylaxis services. *AIDS and Behavior, 25*(5), 1464–1473. https://doi.org/10.1007/s10461-020-02985-0

Ericksen, K. P., & Trocki, K. F. (1992). Behavioral risk factors for sexually transmitted disease in american households. *Social Science & Medicine, 34*(8), 843–853. https://doi.org/10.1016/0277-9536(92)90254-N

Ezell, J. M., Pho, M., Jaiswal, J., Ajayi, B. P., Gosnell, N., Kay, E., Eaton, E., & Bluthenthal, R. (2023). A systematic literature review of strengths-based approaches to drug use management and treatment. *Clinical Social Work Journal, 51*(3), 294–305. https://doi.org/10.1007/s10615-023-00874-2

Ferlatte, O., Salway, T., Oliffe, J. L., & Trussler, T. (2017). Stigma and suicide among gay and bisexual men living with HIV. *AIDS Care, 29*(11), 1346–1350. https://doi.org/10.1080/09540121.2017.1290762

Ferrer, R. A., & Klein, W. M. (2015). Risk perceptions and health behavior. *Current Opinion in Psychology, 5*, 85–89. https://doi.org/10.1016/j.copsyc.2015.03.012

Ford, C. L., & Airhihenbuwa, C. O. (2010). Critical race theory, race equity, and public health: Toward antiracism praxis. *American Journal of Public Health, 100*(S1), S30–S35. https://doi.org/10.2105/AJPH.2009.171058

Friedman, S. R., Mateu-Gelabert, P., Sandoval, M., Hagan, H., & Jarlais, D. C. (2008). Positive deviance control-case life history: A method to develop grounded hypotheses about successful long-term avoidance of infection. *BMC Public Health, 8*(1), 94. https://doi.org/10.1186/1471-2458-8-94

Glick, S. N., Cleary, S. D., & Golden, M. R. (2015). Increasing acceptance of homosexuality in the United States across racial and ethnic subgroups. *Journal of Acquired Immune Deficiency Syndromes, 70*, 319–322. https://doi.org/10.1097/QAI.0000000000000740

Golub, S. A., & Myers, J. E. (2019). Next-wave HIV pre-exposure prophylaxis implementation for gay and bisexual men. *AIDS Patient Care and STDs, 33*(6), 253–261. https://doi.org/10.1089/apc.2018.0290

Grant, J. S., Stafylis, C., Celum, C., Grennan, T., Haire, B., Kaldor, J., Luetkemeyer, A. F., Saunders, J. M., Molina, J.-M., & Klausner, J. D. (2020). Doxycycline prophylaxis for bacterial sexually transmitted infections. *Clinical Infectious Diseases, 70*(6), 1247–1253. https://doi.org/10.1093/cid/ciz866

Hall, K. S. (2012). The health belief model can guide modern contraceptive behavior research and practice. *Journal of Midwifery & Women's Health, 57*(1), 74–81. https://doi.org/10.1111/j.1542-2011.2011.00110.x

Hammack, P. L., & Cohler, B. J. (2011). Narrative, identity, and the politics of exclusion: Social change and the gay and lesbian life course. *Sexuality Research and Social Policy, 8*(3), 162. https://doi.org/10.1007/s13178-011-0060-3

Hammond, W. P., Matthews, D., & Corbie-Smith, G. (2010). Psychosocial factors associated with routine health examination scheduling and receipt among African American men. *Journal of the National Medical Association, 102*(4), 276–289.

Herrick, A. L., Lim, S. H., Wei, C., Smith, H., Guadamuz, T., Friedman, M. S., & Stall, R. (2011). Resilience as an untapped resource in behavioral intervention design for gay men. *AIDS and Behavior, 15*(1), 25–29. https://doi.org/10.1007/s10461-011-9895-0

Herrick, A. L., Stall, R., Goldhammer, H., Egan, J. E., & Mayer, K. H. (2014). Resilience as a research framework and as a cornerstone of prevention research for gay and bisexual men: Theory and evidence. *AIDS and Behavior, 18*(1), 1–9. https://doi.org/10.1007/s10461-012-0384-x

Hess, K. L., Hu, X., Lansky, A., Mermin, J., & Hall, H. I. (2017). Lifetime risk of a diagnosis of HIV infection in the United States. *Annals of Epidemiology, 27*(4), 238–243. https://doi.org/10.1016/j.annepidem.2017.02.003

Hickson, D. A., Truong, N. L., Smith-Bankhead, N., Sturdevant, N., Duncan, D. T., Schnorr, J., Gipson, J. A., & Mena, L. A. (2015). Rationale, design and methods of the ecological study of sexual behaviors and HIV/STI among African American men who have sex with men in the southeastern United States (the MARI study). *PLoS One, 10*(12), e0143823. https://doi.org/10.1371/journal.pone.0143823

Hoffman, K. M., Trawalter, S., Axt, J. R., & Oliver, M. N. (2016). Racial bias in pain assessment and treatment recommendations, and false beliefs about biological differences between blacks and whites. *Proceedings of the National Academy of Sciences, 113*(16), 4296–4301. https://doi.org/10.1073/pnas.1516047113

Hotton, A. L., Balthazar, C., Jadwin-Cakmak, L., Gwiazdowski, B., Castillo, M., Harper, G. W., & Hosek, S. G. (2020). Socio-structural factors associated with mental health, substance use, and HIV risk among Black sexual and gender minorities in the house and ball community. *AIDS and Behavior, 24*, 2319–2326. https://doi.org/10.1007/s10461-020-02791-8

Janz, N. K., & Becker, M. H. (1984). The health belief model: A decade later. *Health Education Quarterly, 11*(1), 1–47. https://doi.org/10.1177/109019818401100101

Johnson, R. L., Roter, D., Powe, N. R., & Cooper, L. A. (2004). Patient race/ethnicity and quality of patient–physician communication during medical visits. *American Journal of Public Health, 94*(12), 2084–2090. https://doi.org/10.2105/AJPH.94.12.2084

Kirby, T. (2020). Cabotegravir, a new option for PrEP. *The Lancet Infectious Diseases, 20*(7), 781. https://doi.org/10.1016/S1473-3099(20)30497-7

Koblin, B. A., Mayer, K. H., Eshleman, S. H., Wang, L., Mannheimer, S., del Rio, C., Shoptaw, S., Magnus, M., Buchbinder, S., Wilton, L., Liu, T.-Y., Cummings, V., Piwowar-Manning, E., Fields, S. D., Griffith, S., Elharrar, V., & Wheeler, D. (2013). Correlates of HIV acquisition in a cohort of Black men who have sex with men in the United States: HIV prevention trials network (HPTN) 061. *PLoS One, 8*(7), e70413. https://doi.org/10.1371/journal.pone.0070413

Koester, K. A., Erguera, X. A., Kang Dufour, M.-S., Udoh, I., Burack, J. H., Grant, R. M., & Myers, J. J. (2018). "Losing the phobia:" understanding how HIV pre-exposure prophylaxis facilitates bridging the serodivide among men who have sex with men. *Frontiers in Public Health, 6*. https://doi.org/10.3389/fpubh.2018.00250

Leichliter, J. S., Dittus, P. J., Copen, C. E., & Aral, S. O. (2020). Trends in factors indicating increased risk for STI among key subpopulations in the United States, 2002–2015. *Sexually Transmitted Infections, 96*(2), 121–123. https://doi.org/10.1136/sextrans-2019-054045

Liboro, R., Despres, J., Ranuschio, B., Bell, S., & Barnes, L. (2021). Forging resilience to HIV/AIDS: Personal strengths of middle-aged and older gay, bisexual, and other men who have sex with men living with HIV/AIDS. *American Journal of Men's Health, 15*(5), 15579883211049016. https://doi.org/10.1177/15579883211049016

Maiman, L. A., & Becker, M. H. (1974). The health belief model: Origins and correlates in psychological theory. *Health Education Monographs, 2*(4), 336–353. https://doi.org/10.1177/109019817400200404

Maina, I. W., Belton, T. D., Ginzberg, S., Singh, A., & Johnson, T. J. (2018). A decade of studying implicit racial/ethnic bias in healthcare providers using the implicit association test. *Social Science & Medicine, 199*, 219–229. https://doi.org/10.1016/j.socscimed.2017.05.009

Mansergh, G., & Marks, G. (1998). Age and risk of HIV infection in men who have sex with men. *AIDS (London, England), 12*(10), 1119–1128.

Markus, H., & Nurius, P. (1986). Possible selves. *American Psychologist, 41*(9), 954–969. https://doi.org/10.1037/0003-066X.41.9.954

Marsh, D. R., Schroeder, D. G., Dearden, K. A., Sternin, J., & Sternin, M. (2004). The power of positive deviance. *BMJ, 329*(7475), 1177–1179. https://doi.org/10.1136/bmj.329.7475.1177

Maulsby, C., Millett, G., Lindsey, K., Kelley, R., Johnson, K., Montoya, D., & Holtgrave, D. (2013). A systematic review of HIV interventions for Black men who have sex with men (MSM). *BMC Public Health, 13*, 625. https://doi.org/10.1186/1471-2458-13-625

Mayer, K. H., Molina, J.-M., Thompson, M. A., Anderson, P. L., Mounzer, K. C., De Wet, J. J., DeJesus, E., Jessen, H., Grant, R. M., Ruane, P. J., Wong, P., Ebrahimi, R., Zhong, L., Mathias, A., Callebaut, C., Collins, S. E., Das, M., McCallister, S., Brainard, D. M., Hare, C. B., et al. (2020). Emtricitabine and tenofovir alafenamide vs emtricitabine and tenofovir disoproxil fumarate for HIV pre-exposure prophylaxis (DISCOVER): Primary results from a randomised, double-blind, multicentre, active-controlled, phase 3, non-inferiority trial. *The Lancet, 396*(10246), 239–254. https://doi.org/10.1016/S0140-6736(20)31065-5

McNair, O. S., Gipson, J. A., Denson, D., Thompson, D. V., Sutton, M. Y., & Hickson, D. A. (2018). The associations of resilience and HIV risk behaviors among Black gay, bisexual, and other men who have sex with men (MSM) in the deep south: The MARI study. *AIDS and Behavior, 22*(5), 1679–1687. https://doi.org/10.1007/s10461-017-1881-8

Meyer, I. H. (2007). Prejudice, social stress, and mental health in lesbian, gay, and bisexual populations. *Conceptual Issues and Research Evidence, 39*.

Millett, G. A., Flores, S. A., Peterson, J. L., & Bakeman, R. (2007). Explaining disparities in HIV infection among Black and white men who have sex with men: A meta-analysis of HIV risk behaviors. *AIDS, 21*(15), 2083–2091. https://doi.org/10.1097/QAD.0b013e3282e9a64b

Millett, G. A., Peterson, J. L., Flores, S. A., Hart, T. A., Jeffries, W. L., 4th, Wilson, P. A., Rourke, S. B., Heilig, C. M., Elford, J., Fenton, K. A., & Remis, R. S. (2012). Comparisons of disparities and risks of HIV infection in Black and other men who have sex with men in Canada, UK, and USA: A meta-analysis. *The Lancet, 380*(9839), 341–348. https://doi.org/10.1016/S0140-6736(12)60899-X

Mustanski, B., Newcomb, M. E., & Clerkin, E. M. (2011). Relationship characteristics and sexual risk-taking in young men who have sex with men. *Health Psychology, 30*(5), 597–605. https://doi.org/10.1037/a0023858

National Institute of Allergy and Infectious Diseases. (2019, May 21). *HIV Undetectable=Untransmittable (U=U), or Treatment as Prevention.* https://www.niaid.nih.gov/diseases-conditions/treatment-prevention

Nelson, K. M., Gamarel, K. E., Pantalone, D. W., Carey, M. P., & Simoni, J. M. (2016). Sexual debut and HIV-related sexual risk-taking by birth cohort among men who have sex with men in the United States. *AIDS and Behavior, 20*(10), 2286–2295. https://doi.org/10.1007/s10461-016-1330-0

Ober, A. J., Dangerfield, D. T., Shoptaw, S., Ryan, G., Stucky, B., & Friedman, S. R. (2018). Using a "positive deviance" framework to discover adaptive risk reduction behaviors among high-risk HIV negative Black men who have sex with men. *AIDS and Behavior, 22*(5), 1699–1712. https://doi.org/10.1007/s10461-017-1790-x

Osmond, D. H., Pollack, L. M., Paul, J. P., & Catania, J. A. (2007). Changes in prevalence of HIV infection and sexual risk behavior in men who have sex with men in San Francisco: 1997 2002. *American Journal of Public Health, 97*(9), 1677–1683. https://doi.org/10.2105/AJPH.2005.062851

Oyserman, D., Terry, K., & Bybee, D. (2002). A possible selves intervention to enhance school involvement. *Journal of Adolescence, 25*(3), 313–326. https://doi.org/10.1006/jado.2002.0474

Oyserman, D., Bybee, D., & Terry, K. (2006). Possible selves and academic outcomes: How and when possible selves impel action. *Journal of Personality and Social Psychology, 91*(1), 188–204. https://doi.org/10.1037/0022-3514.91.1.188

Pinto, R. M., Berringer, K. R., Melendez, R., & Mmeje, O. (2018). Improving PrEP implementation through multilevel interventions: A synthesis of the literature. *AIDS and Behavior, 22*(11), 3681–3691. https://doi.org/10.1007/s10461-018-2184-4

Poteat, T. C., & Logie, C. H. (2022). A case for strengths-based approaches to addressing intersectional stigma in HIV research. *American Journal of Public Health, 112*(S4), S347–S349. https://doi.org/10.2105/AJPH.2021.306659

Quinn, K. G., & Voisin, D. R. (2020). ART adherence among men who have sex with men living with HIV: Key challenges and opportunities. *Current HIV/AIDS Reports, 17*, 290–300. https://doi.org/10.1007/s11904-020-00510-5

Quinn, K., Voisin, D. R., Bouris, A., & Schneider, J. (2016). Psychological distress, drug use, sexual risks and medication adherence among young HIV-positive Black men who have sex with men: Exposure to community violence matters. *AIDS Care, 28*(7), 866–872. https://doi.org/10.1080/09540121.2016.1153596

Quinn, K., Dickson-Gomez, J., Zarwell, M., Pearson, B., & Lewis, M. (2018). "A gay man and a doctor are just like, a recipe for destruction": How racism and homonegativity in healthcare settings influence PrEP uptake among young Black MSM. *AIDS and Behavior, 23*, 1951–1963. https://doi.org/10.1007/s10461-018-2375-z

Quinn, K., Bowleg, L., & Dickson-Gomez, J. (2019). "The fear of being Black plus the fear of being gay": The effects of intersectional stigma on PrEP use among young Black gay, bisexual, and other men who have sex with men. *Social Science & Medicine, 232*, 86–93. https://doi.org/10.1016/j.socscimed.2019.04.042

Randolph, S. D., Golin, C., Welgus, H., Lightfoot, A. F., Harding, C. J., & Riggins, L. F. (2020). How perceived structural racism and discrimination and medical mistrust in the health system influences participation in HIV health services for Black women living in the United States South: A qualitative, descriptive study. *Journal of the Association of Nurses in AIDS Care, 31*(5), 598–605. https://doi.org/10.1097/JNC.0000000000000189

Rhodes, T. (2002). The 'risk environment': A framework for understanding and reducing drug-related harm. *International Journal of Drug Policy, 13*(2), 85–94. https://doi.org/10.1016/S0955-3959(02)00007-5

Risher, K., Mayer, K., & Beyrer, C. (2015). The HIV treatment cascade in men who have sex with men, people who inject drugs and sex workers. *Current Opinion in HIV and AIDS, 10*(6), 420–429. https://doi.org/10.1097/COH.0000000000000200

Rosenstock, I. M. (1974a). Historical origins of the health belief model. *Health Education Monographs, 2*(4), 328–335. https://doi.org/10.1177/109019817400200403

Rosenstock, I. M. (1974b). The health belief model and preventive health behavior. *Health Education Monographs, 2*(4), 354–386. https://doi.org/10.1177/109019817400200405

Rosenstock, I. M., Strecher, V. J., & Becker, M. H. (1994). The health belief model and HIV risk behavior change. In R. J. DiClemente & J. L. Peterson (Eds.), *Preventing AIDS: Theories and methods of behavioral interventions* (pp. 5–24). Springer US. https://doi.org/10.1007/978-1-4899-1193-3_2

Rothman, K. J., Greenland, S., & Lash, T. L. (2008). *Modern epidemiology*. Lippincott Williams & Wilkins.

Shen, M. J., Peterson, E. B., Costas-Muñiz, R., Hernandez, M. H., Jewell, S. T., Matsoukas, K., & Bylund, C. L. (2018). The effects of race and racial concordance on patient-physician communication: A systematic review of the literature. *Journal of Racial and Ethnic Health Disparities, 5*(1), 117–140. https://doi.org/10.1007/s40615-017-0350-4

Sullivan, P. S., Peterson, J., Rosenberg, E. S., Kelley, C. F., Cooper, H., Vaughan, A., Salazar, L. F., Frew, P., Wingood, G., DiClemente, R., del Rio, C., Mulligan, M., & Sanchez, T. H. (2014). Understanding racial HIV/STI disparities in Black and white men who have sex with men: A multilevel approach. *PLoS One, 9*(3), e90514. https://doi.org/10.1371/journal.pone.0090514

Sullivan, P. S., Mena, L., Elopre, L., & Siegler, A. J. (2019). Implementation strategies to increase PrEP uptake in the south. *Current HIV/AIDS Reports, 16*(4), 259–269. https://doi.org/10.1007/s11904-019-00447-4

Sullivan, P. S., Knox, J., Jones, J., Taussig, J., Graves, M. V., Millett, G., Luisi, N., Hall, E., Sanchez, T. H., Rio, C. D., Kelley, C., Rosenberg, E. S., & Guest, J. L. (2021). Understanding disparities in viral suppression among Black MSM living with HIV in Atlanta Georgia. *Journal of the International AIDS Society, 24*(4), e25689. https://doi.org/10.1002/jia2.25689

US Food and Drug Administration. (2021, December 20). *FDA approves first injectable treatment for HIV pre-exposure prevention*. FDA. https://www.fda.gov/news-events/press-announcements/fda-approves-first-injectable-treatment-hiv-pre-exposure-prevention

Voisin, D. R., Quinn, K., Kim, D. H., & Schneider, J. (2017). A longitudinal analysis of antiretroviral adherence among young Black men who have sex with men. *Journal of Adolescent Health, 60*(4), 411–416. https://doi.org/10.1016/j.jadohealth.2016.10.428

von Hippel, C. (2018). A next generation assets-based public health intervention development model: The public as innovators. *Frontiers in Public Health, 6*, 248. https://doi.org/10.3389/fpubh.2018.00248

Winder, T. J. A., & Lea, C. H. (2019). “Blocking” and “filtering”: A commentary on mobile technology, racism, and the sexual networks of young Black MSM (YBMSM). *Journal of Racial and Ethnic Health Disparities, 6*(2), 231–236. https://doi.org/10.1007/s40615-018-0493-y

Chapter 3
Recruiting, Retaining, and Engaging Black Sexual Minority Men in HIV/STI Prevention Research

Chapter Objectives

1. Identify the barriers and facilitators of prevention research engagement among Black sexual minority men (SMM).
2. Describe effective protocols, techniques, and strategies to engage Black SMM in HIV/STI prevention research
3. Explore ethical considerations for targeted community engagement

The Importance of Intentional Recruitment and Community Engagement Protocols

Intentional community engagement and study recruitment is crucial for prevention science with Black SMM for several reasons. First, it ensures that recruitment protocols are effective and enable researchers to study a diverse sample that represents the population; obtaining a diverse sample is essential for generalizing the study findings to the broader community. Intentional recruitment protocols also substantially affect the quality of data collection. Properly planning and executing recruitment and retention protocols can prevent study delays and reduce the costs (financial and professional) associated with extended research timelines. Moreover, fair recruitment activities build trust from the community and encourages individuals to participate in future studies, which is key for the long-term sustainability of research programs.

Despite the challenges generally faced in recruiting and retaining Black SMM for sexual health research, my studies have consistently seen high participation and retention from the community. Additionally, participants have openly shared highly

D. T. Dangerfield II, *Prevention Science & Targeted Methods for HIV/STI Research with Black Sexual Minority Men*,
https://doi.org/10.1007/978-3-031-85130-8_3

sensitive information regarding their sexuality, experiences with trauma, and substance use in my studies (Dangerfield II et al., 2017, 2020, 2022b), which is crucial to obtaining necessary data for identifying community needs and designing relevant interventions. This provides hope for prevention scientists to engage highly apprehensive community members and learn key information to support public health activities. However, careful consideration to recruitment and community engagement protocols is needed to build trust, improve research participation interest, and obtain full disclosure from study participants. Therefore, this chapter outlines protocols, techniques, and strategies to effectively recruit, retain, and engage this Black SMM in sexual health prevention research. These approaches can help prevention scientists (and other researchers) build trust and obtain diverse samples from a marginalized and often apprehensive community, which is essential for targeted sexual health prevention research.

Understanding the Barriers to Research Engagement Among Black Sexual Minority Men

Overall, recruiting Black SMM for research studies involves several challenges that reflect broader social issues of trust, stigma, and access. For example, there is substantial mistrust of medical and research institutions partly due to historical abuses in Black communities from violence and deception in research studies such as the Tuskegee Syphilis Study (Dangerfield II & Wylie, 2022; Scharff et al., 2010). This mistrust has extended into contemporary research participation as some Black SMM fear mistreatment, exploitation, privacy breaches, or misuse of personal information (Dangerfield II et al., 2021b, 2022a). The oversaturation of targeted, HIV-focused research and interventions among Black SMM also exacerbates their skepticism and concerns about further stigmatization (Calabrese et al., 2023). Their individual experiences of racism, discrimination, and stigma from society, clinicians, and researchers also exacerbate the background mistrust of research and reduces willingness to participate in studies (Scharff et al., 2010; White et al., 2019). Some believe that their experiences and perspectives regarding race, sexuality, and adversity are generally ignored and misunderstood by researchers and clinicians (Cahill et al., 2017; Dangerfield II et al., 2022a; Quinn et al., 2018). Therefore, some community members are reluctant to participate in sexual health studies without attention or acknowledgement of other important social issues in their lives.

Added to this, socio-economic factors including limited access to transportation and inflexible work hours can also affect recruitment and research participation among Black SMM. Studies that require frequent visits or lengthy participation might be less accessible or attractive to individuals who cannot afford to take time off from work or travel (Dangerfield II & Wylie, 2022). STI/HIV prevention studies usually enroll low-resourced participants partly because study appointment times are typically during normal business hours when professionals are working and study incentives are unattractive to middle class individuals. Some participants also perceive typical gift card incentives ($25–$50) as unfair or inequitable for their participation in clinical studies given the amount of data being collected for typical sexual health studies (Dangerfield II & Wylie, 2022). Studies will not obtain diverse samples of Black SMM unless attention is paid to these socio-economic, historical, and cultural issues. To ensure more inclusive recruitment, researchers must consider alternative strategies, such as offering flexible scheduling, providing transportation assistance, or increasing the value of incentives to better reflect participants' time and effort. Engaging with popular opinion leaders, gatekeepers, and community organizations can help build trust and facilitate participation among Black SMM.

Building Research Teams Before Recruitment Starts

In some geographic and cultural contexts, such as the U.S. South, homosexuality is heavily stigmatized and supportive organizations are few. Additionally, some community members will not participate in a research study unless an in-group member or popular opinion leader has endorsed it. Therefore, partnerships with gatekeepers are required to access the community because it is "hidden" or marginalized from traditional spaces. Gatekeepers are individuals or organizations that have direct access to potential research participants. They could be community leaders, popular clinicians, healthcare administrators, or the heads of social groups (e.g., a "House Mother"). Gatekeepers help ensure that the recruitment process and study protocols are ethical and equitable for the community. They might also assess whether the researchers and the proposed study respects cultural sensitivities and addresses community needs. Their endorsement and approval are necessary for researchers to access and recruit target communities. Establishing genuine partnerships with local gatekeepers, clinics, and/or community-based organizations is key to receiving endorsements from individuals who could recommend community members to participate in the study. These partnerships can help build trust in the research team and study aims, provide direct referrals to others, and invite researchers to attend social spaces where they can build rapport with the community (and potentially recruit for the study). Having rapport with the community can help increase the number of referrals to the study and effectively recruiting Black SMM. Moreover, collaborating with the community provides additional opportunities to learn more about their needs for culturally responsive solutions. Ultimately, adopting these strategies is essential for fostering equitable research practices that not only enhance study validity but also contribute to the empowerment and well-being of Black SMM communities.

Real Academic-Community Partnerships

Building a collaborative relationship (and trust) with the community is similar to any other relationship. Researchers should show genuine interest in the community and the work of gatekeepers and build rapport *before* they need something (i.e., help with recruitment). Black SMM have consistently shared that they want researchers to demonstrate care for the overall health and wellness of the community and not just recruit them for studies (Dangerfield II et al., 2021a, 2022a; Dangerfield II & Wylie, 2022). The partnership can take on different forms. In my work, I have volunteered in several capacities at community-based organizations globally to build trust, demonstrate my commitment, and learn more about community needs. For example, I have joined community health workers on mobile units to help recruit individuals for HIV/STI testing in the field, presented research for community-based organizations, and analyzed clinic data for organization reports. The goal is to identify ways in which your presence as a researcher can be helpful to the organization in the absence of your research goals. Researchers who invest time and effort into serving organizations may be more likely to receive endorsements from gatekeepers and key stakeholders who will refer the community to screen for your study. Therefore, it is crucial to find equitable opportunities for researchers to support gatekeepers, build trust, and gain a better understanding of the needs and interests of the community.

Matching Researcher Preferences of the Community

Given the background mistrust, apprehension, and marginalization of the community, effective engagement with Black SMM in research generally necessitates the inclusion of prevention scientists who are from the community and a significant investment of time and effort. Having study team members who are part of the target population is crucial for gaining access, generating sufficient samples, and facilitating research participation with minority populations. Additionally, investing intensive time and effort is essential for obtaining valid data because some Black SMM will not disclose the full range of their behaviors, attitudes, and experiences to non-Black researchers (Dangerfield II et al., 2018, 2022a; White et al., 2019). Socially marginalized individuals often feel more comfortable and understood by research teams that reflect their community. National data from the Pew Research Center showed that Blacks are more receptive to science and medicine when they see successful Black people in the field (Funk, 2022). Some will not participate or discuss the full range of their experiences, attitudes, or behaviors to researchers who are not racial or sexual minorities, which limits the field's ability to generate solutions for the community. My research identified how some Black SMM believe Black researchers would provide better care and interpret the findings of clinical studies than non-Black researchers partly because they believe that Black researchers have greater investment in the overall wellness of the community. In a focus group study published in *JMIR Human Factors* (Dangerfield II & Wylie, 2022), Black SMM agreed with this man who said,

> We need to see more black queer men doing these research studies, and not necessarily the face of it but actually running them from the start also. So don't just put a Black face on there for image purposes or recruitment purposes, but actually have someone like us running the whole damn thing…In order for me to trust you, I have to feel like you have walked similar spaces that I have. So therefore, you understand where I'm coming from when I'm telling you all this information about it.

Others explicitly say things such as "'*those people' don't really care about us*" and are unwilling to share the full scope of their behaviors and perspectives to non-Black researchers (Dangerfield II & Wylie, 2022; Dangerfield II et al., 2022a; White et al., 2019). Having study team members who are members of the community improves study enrollment regardless of barriers of institutional (i.e., medical and research) mistrust (Magnus et al., 2014; White et al., 2019).

Some researchers and clinicians have explicitly asked me "how do we build the capacity of non-Black researchers to better engage the community?" I have systematically asked Black SMM this question in research studies, to which they reply:

> I feel like it's the wrong question to ask, "how can we get Black folks to trust these white researchers to come and [laughter] get their personal health information?" I think the question really should be, "how can we find more Black researchers? And how can we get more Black doctors? And how can we set them up for success in areas where they're able to actually reach out with their community?" The solution is not necessarily to place white doctors in Black communities. That's an extra barrier. And as a researcher, I don't know why you would wanna do that (Dangerfield II & Wylie, 2022).

When possible, culturally equivalent researchers should lead research and recruitment protocols for Black SMM. However, there are still racial and cultural gaps in the leadership of federally sponsored research studies (Hoppe et al., 2019). The underrepresentation of Black SMM in research leadership can lead to a lack of culturally competent recruitment approaches, invalid data, and/or misinterpretation of findings. Therefore, sexual health prevention research may be missing an important proportion of the community that is apprehensive about research participation if studies are not led by similar scientists. Research teams must include culturally similar scientists to build credibility in the research and engage in a combination of active and passive strategies to enhance recruitment, retention, and community engagement. Ultimately, the culture of the research teams should reflect an understanding of the dynamics within the community to build trust that prevention scientists have an investment in the community's needs and can interpret and articulate findings correctly.

Community-Based Versus Community-Placed Research

One way to build trust, engage the community, and enhance scientific capacity for accurate results interpretation is by involving the community in the research process. However, there are inconsistencies in the degree of community engagement and in how these approaches are categorized in sexual health prevention science. These inconsistencies can result in varying levels of participant involvement, effectiveness in addressing community-specific issues, and trust, especially if researchers misclassify their methods. To address this, it is essential to review the various forms of community-engaged research to identify and establish best practices for sexual health prevention science. Clarifying the language and approaches of these practices will help ensure more consistent methodological understandings, ultimately improving the impact and relevance of research outcomes.

Community-based research takes community involvement to a higher level by establishing a collaborative partnership between researchers and community members throughout the entire research process. Community-based research generally values the perspectives, knowledge, and experiences of those directly impacted by the issues being studied and ensures that these are incorporated as the community of interest actively helps identify problems and develop solutions (Israel et al., 1998). This approach ensures that the research addresses the community's needs and leverages local knowledge in the science, leading to more relevant and effective outcomes. Community-based participatory research (CBPR) emphasizes co-learning, mutual respect, and shared decision-making (Israel et al., 1998, 2010). The partnership in CBPR is characterized by equity and empowerment, fostering a sense of research ownership among community members. Ultimately, community-based research bridges the gap between academic research and real-world practice, contributing to more effective and equitable health and social outcomes. This collaborative effort enhances the validity and applicability of research findings and facilitates the implementation of interventions that are culturally sensitive and sustainable. However, some prevention research studies may claim that the approach is community-based, but should be reclassified as "community-placed" because it lacks complete partnership and does not fully engage the voices of the community throughout the research process. In these cases, the community's role is often limited to a passive recipient of interventions or data collection sites rather than an active collaborator in shaping the research agenda, design, and implementation. This superficial engagement could undermine the effectiveness and sustainability of interventions, as they may not fully reflect the community's priorities, needs, or cultural context. True community-based research requires a deeper commitment to shared power, trust-building, and continuous dialogue, ensuring that the community's voice is integral to every stage of the research process.

"Community-placed research," as far as I see it, refers to studies conducted within a community setting but without substantial involvement or collaboration with community members in the research process. In community-placed research, prevention scientists typically design and implement the study independently, using "the community" as a location for data collection rather than as active partners. This approach can be useful for gathering data on general populations and can provide trusted contexts for data collection. However, it often misses the nuanced understanding and contextual insights that come from engaging vulnverable subpopulations, especially if the study is not led by scientists who are from the target population or community context. Although this approach can still build trust and yield important data by being conducted in settings that are familiar to participants, this top-down methodology can overlook local priorities and fail to address community-specific needs. Moreover, the lack of community involvement can lead to mistrust or a feeling of being exploited among community members. The lack of community involvement can lead to mistrust or a feeling of being exploited among community members, as they may perceive the research as something being done *to* them rather than *with* them. This can undermine the long-term success of interventions and reduce the likelihood that the findings will be translated into meaningful, sustainable change. Ultimately, while community-placed research can offer valuable insights, it falls short of the transformative potential of CBPR, which fosters true collaboration, empowers communities, and ensures that research outcomes are relevant, equitable, and impactful.

Active Recruitment Strategies

Active recruitment refers to direct interactions with the target community whereby the study team provides information to interested individuals. For example, active recruitment can involve the following approaches:

- Attending LGBT-friendly bars, clubs, or outreach events and discussing the study with interested individuals in the field.
- Reaching out to participants from previous studies who provided consent to be contacted for future research.
- Reviewing records from the medical information management system (with IRB and organizational approval) of clinics and community-based organizations to screen patients for eligibility and inviting them to participate in the study using patient portals.

The goal of active recruitment is for the study team to be visible to community members and provide as much information about the study as efficiently and comprehensibly as possible. To achieve this, study team members can engage in active recruitment at bars and clubs on a regular basis, ensuring a consistent presence in locations where potential participants are likely to gather. Additionally, they should attend community-based events as relevant activities arise throughout the year, such as festivals, health fairs, and meetings at community support groups. By doing so, the study team can build rapport and trust with community members, making them more likely to consider participating in the study. Moreover, these interactions provide opportunities to address any questions or concerns directly, further enhancing understanding and interest in the research. Effective active recruitment strategies can significantly increase participation rates and ensure a diverse and representative sample for the study. Of note, Black SMM have suggested that researchers who are not Black and/or gay should socialize with the community at events and places where they frequent to build rapport (and trust) and mitigate medical/research mistrust (Dangerfield II et al., 2021a; Dangerfield II & Wylie, 2022). More research is needed to explore the ethical, professional, and enrollment implications of researchers targeting places where Black gay and bisexual men frequent for social activities.

Passive Recruitment Strategies

Passive study recruitment strategies are generally less direct than active methods but can still be highly effective, especially in reaching a broad audience. In passive study recruitment, potential participants are not actively approached by researchers. Instead, the information about the study is made available through various channels and interested individuals must contact the researchers to learn more about the study and screen for participation. Passive recruitment strategies might include the following activities:

- Posting flyers or posters in community centers, clinics, or universities
- Online advertising on social media, geosocial networking apps, websites, or newsletters
- Placing advertisements on public transit
- Referrals from peers, social networks, or individuals who previously participated in the study (snowball sampling)

Passive recruitment can be used to help ensure that the recruitment process is less biased and that participants voluntarily express interest, which can help maintain ethical standards in research. Passive recruitment methods are also often less costly because they can save on personnel costs and can continuously attract participants without the need for direct interaction. Using online advertisements on location-based platforms help researchers reach marginalized populations better than time-venue recruitment activities (Wei et al., 2012). However, they require well-thought-out materials that respect and reflect the cultural and individual diversity of the target population to be effective. My experience recruiting Black SMM for studies in Maryland and Washington, D.C. suggests that geosocial networking apps can reach ~500 SMM in about 2 weeks, depending on the nature of the study (it is important note that all of these individuals might not be eligible). Passive recruitment strategies such as word of mouth or snowball sampling can also engage marginalized communities better than true random sampling, which is often not feasible for research with racial and sexual minority men (Wei et al., 2012). Incorporating culturally sensitive and inclusive materials into passive recruitment strategies is essential for effectively engaging marginalized communities and ensuring that research participation is both voluntary and representative.

Retention and Study Engagement

Once a study has recruited eligible volunteers to participate, ensuring that they remain in the study and engage fully are important for success. The key to retention is building respect and trust between the research team and the study participants. Regular communication and personalized interactions play a crucial role in maintaining this trust and engagement (Dangerfield II et al., 2021b; White et al., 2019). Researchers should collect detailed tracking information (e.g., mailing address, email, phone number, social media information, and additional contact person) using an IRB-approved Future Contact form. This information is used to locate participants who miss appointments for rescheduling. This information is also used to conduct wellness phone calls and send monthly greeting cards (handwritten notes or electronic cards) during interim visits to maintain rapport with participants. In my research protocols, the study team typically communicates with participants at least twice prior to focus group participation to clarify the study objectives and remind interested participants of focus group meeting times. This has contributed to the our ability to conduct most of our focus groups with at least five Black SMM within 8 weeks (Dangerfield II et al., 2021b; White et al., 2019). Targeted data show that these interactions during interim visits demonstrate "care" and investment in the overall health of Black SMM (Dangerfield II et al., 2021a; Dangerfield II & Wylie, 2022). Additionally, post-group follow-up calls to express appreciation and gather feedback help maintain community interest and foster a sense of study ownership. This genuine approach not only improves retention rates but also enhances the quality and relevance of the data collected. It also improves willingness for individuals to participate in future studies.

Conducting Studies at Preferred Venues

Despite general protections, guidance, and regulations from IRB regarding study conduct, some eligible individuals do not maintain their appointments for studies that are conducted on campus at academic institutions because of the history of medical research mistreatment in Black communities (White et al., 2019). Therefore, being intentional and considerate about where studies are conducted is also key to protecting human subjects (Happell, 2007). Conducting research studies in venues where participants feel comfortable is crucial when considering recruitment, engagement, and retention because their experiences of mistreatment and marginalization exacerbate their unwillingness to participate in studies. Black SMM must be in environments where their privacy is protected and their safety is prioritized. Researchers should identify study settings where participants feel comfortable and that they feel that their privacy is protected to improve their willingness to share information. These venues can include community-based organizations, clinic office spaces, hotel conference rooms (for focus groups), or virtually on Zoom

(Dangerfield II et al., 2021b; White et al., 2019). Qualitative approaches such as focus groups should provide multiple location options, one of which should include a community-based location and the other should explore the preferences for study location then the groups should be conducted at a location agreed upon by focus group members. Organizing the preferences of eligible volunteers can be labor intensive for the research team but will likely establish more trust and participation from study participants.

Study Incentives and Participant Remuneration

Incentives play a crucial role in the success of prevention research by motivating participants to engage and complete the study. They can substantially enhance recruitment and retention rates, which ensures a diverse and representative sample, and encourage full participation. Incentives can also suggest how much the researchers value the contribution of participants. By offering incentives such as monetary compensation, gift cards, or other benefits (e.g., health screenings, experimental treatments), researchers can encourage higher levels of participation and commitment from eligible volunteers. This, in turn, can improve data quality and validity because participants might be more likely to follow through with the study's requirements. Moreover, thoughtful incentives can foster a positive relationship between researchers and participants, promoting trust and encouraging future participation in studies by your team.

Since medical and research mistrust persists for Black SMM, immediately incentivizing participants after their study participation is crucial to limit mistrust and skepticism. However, administrative barriers can cause delays in participant incentives. In my work, administrative challenges have caused individuals to reach out to the institution and make formal complaints about not receiving timely incentives for their participation. For example, two participants in one of my studies reached out to the IRB with concerns that the research team was taking advantage of their participation and did not believe that the study would compensate them for their time. This caused us to identify ways to immediately incentivize participants after their participation, especially for virtual studies (Dangerfield II et al., 2021b). Ultimately, administrative regulations on virtual incentives were updated and we were able to promptly disburse claim codes electronically when participants completed their study visit. However, it is important that research institutions continually review and streamline incentive distribution processes to ensure timely compensation, maintain participant trust, and address any emerging administrative challenges. This ongoing effort not only upholds ethical standards but also fosters a positive relationship between researchers and participants, encouraging continued engagement and participation in future studies.

It is also important to balance the use of incentives with ethical considerations to avoid coercion. Coercion occurs when participants feel pressured to join or remain in a study due to the offered incentives, potentially compromising their voluntary consent. To prevent this, researchers should ensure that incentives are appropriate and proportionate to the time and effort required by the study, and clearly communicate that participation is entirely voluntary. This careful balance helps maintain ethical standards while still encouraging meaningful participation. High cash incentives are often considered coercive because they can exert undue influence on individuals to participate in studies, leading them to make decisions during the study (including participating in the first place) that they might not otherwise consider.

Offering large sums of money can raise ethical concerns, especially in contexts such as medical trials or employment. When the financial incentive is substantially high, although there is no consensus as to what amount is considered "high", individuals might feel pressured to participate due to their financial needs rather than their genuine interest or willingness. This can compromise the true voluntary nature of their consent. Some individuals may agree to participate in activities or decisions that they wouldn't consider under normal circumstances because they need the money. The concern is that individuals might overlook potential risks or personal reservations due to the attractiveness of the financial reward. Therefore, high incentives can create a power imbalance between scientists and the participant, which can lead to situations where the recipient feels they have no choice but to accept the offer, even if it is not in their best interest. These factors contribute to the perception that high cash incentives can be coercive, as they might unduly influence individuals' decisions, undermining the principles of voluntary and informed consent.

How much of an Incentive Should Participants Receive?

Study incentives range depending upon the nature of the study. Most HIV prevention studies offer ~$25 gift card incentives for participation. In my studies, cash incentives ranging from $40–$80 are provided as often as possible. In most of our studies, which have involved one-time interviews, focus groups, or surveys, participants who refer other eligible volunteers are compensated an additional $40 electronic gift card for each eligible volunteer they referred up to two referrals. The quarantine of 2020 prevented in-person protocols and our studies subsequently provided $75–$80 electronic Amazon gift cards as incentives. When asked if providing larger cash incentives was coercive, participants across all the groups believed that cash incentives were more equitable for their time and participation in the study (Dangerfield II & Wylie, 2022) by carefully calibrating incentives to reflect the demands of the study without being excessive, researchers can ethically encourage participation while safeguarding participants' autonomy and ensuring their consent is genuinely voluntary. It is crucial for research ethics committees to review incentive plans to strike this delicate balance, ensuring that participants are fairly compensated without feeling coerced.

Informed Consent

Concerns about the adequacy and clarity of informed consent forms are significant for Black SMM and highlight a need for greater transparency and attention to detail in these documents. I have conducted targeted studies examining perceptions of information in informed consent on research trust and participation willingness among Black SMM and found that despite information describing how a consent form would detail the risks and privacy measures involved, Black SMM perceive typical informed consent documents to be insufficient to build their trust in the science. Specifically, they do not believe that all known side effects regarding experimental drugs are sufficiently outlined in a consent form and suggested that informed consent forms should explicitly outline intentions not to cause harm participants (Dangerfield II & Wylie, 2022). For example, according to Black SMM, the consent form should include words such as "*Please,*" "*Thank you,*" and "*I will not hurt you,*" providing an example of "care" for participants that researchers should demonstrate.

Regarding data privacy, some men over age 30 suggest that consent forms should further describe "Who really gets access to my data?" They believe that their survey data and health history could be easily obtained by other researchers, clinicians, or pharmaceutical companies who are not a part of the study team. Sometimes a consent form explicitly mentions that data can be used by other researchers who are not a part of the study team, especially when researchers obtain approval to study de-identified data for secondary analyses. Still, this concern reflects background anxiety about the potential misuse of data for purposes beyond the scope of the original study, which has largely been unaddressed by the scientific community. In targeted studies and in community engagement discussions, Black SMM emphasize the importance of clear, specific language in consent forms that not only identifies who will have access to their data but also explains how it will be protected, stored, and ultimately disposed of. They call for assurances that their information would not be shared with third parties without their knowledge or permission, and suggested that the consent forms include detailed descriptions of data security measures, such as encryption and anonymization, to help alleviate these concerns. Given the ability for secondary research conduct, this may not necessarily be feasible because we do not always know who will request access to data. However, researchers and institutions shuold strive to implement robust data governance policies that balance participant privacy with the potential benefits of future studies. This might include require more rigorous ethical review for second data access, establishing (and evaluating) strict de-identification protocols, and providing participants with transparent explanations of how their data might be used in the future. Although absolute guaranteers of confidentiality are challenging, proactive measures and full disclosures can help build trust and ensure that ethical principles remain central to data-sharing practices. There remains a critical need for researchers to prioritize transparency, cultural sensitivity, and clarity in the development of informed consent documents for Black SMM. Ensuring that consent forms are not only informative but also resonate with the values and expectations of Black SMM is essential for enhancing their willingness to participate in research and for the ethical conduct of studies that aim to address community health issues.

Innovations in Recruitment

Utilizing Facebook groups, social media platforms, and social media influencers presents innovative recruitment strategies to engage Black SMM in prevention research. Facebook groups provide a space where community members already congregate, allowing researchers to connect directly with a targeted audience in a familiar and trusted environment. Social media platforms, such as Instagram and Twitter, enable researchers to reach a broader audience through tailored advertisements and engaging content that resonates with the community's interests and experiences. Collaborating with social media influencers who have a strong following among Black SMM men can further enhance recruitment efforts (Fahey et al., 2024; Pöyry et al., 2022). These influencers can share information about the study, endorse its importance, and encourage their followers to participate, leveraging their credibility and personal connection with their audience. Integrating these digital strategies can help researchers foster a more inclusive and effective recruitment process, greater participation and representation in studies to support the diverse community of Black SMM.

Conclusions

Well-designed recruitment protocols are fundamental to conducting ethical, valid, reliable, and effective research. Addressing recruitment challenges requires thoughtful, culturally sensitive approaches, including having Black SMM research team members, utilizing community-based protocols, training research staff, and providing clear, transparent communication about the purposes and uses of the research. Establishing genuine partnerships with local gatekeepers, clinics, and/or community-based organizations is key to receiving endorsements from individuals who could recommend community members to participate in the study. There is a need for research approaches that are culturally competent and sensitive to the unique experiences of Black SMM. Incentivizing participants in fair and timely ways is crucial to limiting mistrust and skepticism despite the presence of a culturally congruent team. The social challenges that contribute to the sexual health vulnerabilities also impact their willingness and capacity to participate in research studies. Studies must consider cultural nuances and provide a safe, respectful environment that acknowledges their identities and experiences. Training researchers and recruiters in cultural competency, sensitivity, and the specific needs of Black SMM can improve interactions and outcomes in recruitment efforts.

Raised Questions

1. How can researchers ensure that recruitment strategies are culturally sensitive and respectful to the unique experiences of Black SMM?
2. What are the most effective methods for reaching and engaging minority men in health research without compromising their privacy or trust?
3. How can researchers measure and mitigate the impact of potential issues such as selection bias or the influence of socio-economic factors that might arise during recruitment?

Chapter Summary

This chapter delves into the challenges and strategies associated with recruiting, retaining, and engaging Black SMM in HIV/STI prevention research. The chapter outlined the barriers to research participation among Black SMM, including historical mistrust, socio-economic challenges, and the oversaturation of HIV-focused research within this community. It emphasized the importance of intentional recruitment and community engagement protocols, which are crucial for ensuring diverse, representative samples and building trust with participants. The chapter explored both active and passive recruitment strategies, highlighting the need for culturally sensitive approaches that resonate with the target population. It also discussed the role of community partnerships, particularly with gatekeepers, in facilitating access to hidden or marginalized communities and emphasizes the value of building rapport with community members before recruitment begins. Retention and engagement are addressed through strategies such as maintaining regular communication, conducting studies in preferred venues, and offering appropriate incentives. The chapter underscored the importance of informed consent, noting that clarity, transparency, and cultural sensitivity are essential to building trust and ensuring ethical research practices. Innovative recruitment methods, including the use of social media platforms and collaborations with influencers, were presented as effective ways to reach Black SMM. The chapter concluded by advocating for research teams that reflect the cultural and social dynamics of the community, which is crucial for obtaining valid data and fostering long-term engagement in prevention research.

Key Points

1. **Barriers to research engagement among Black SMM**: Black SMM face significant barriers to research participation, including background medical mistrust due to past abuses like the Tuskegee Syphilis Study, current experiences of prejudice and stigma, and the oversaturation of HIV-focused research. These

factors lead to skepticism and a reluctance to engage in studies without attention to broader social issues affecting their lives.

2. **The importance of intentional recruitment and community engagement**: Intentional recruitment and community engagement are crucial for obtaining diverse, representative samples and building trust with Black SMM. Effective recruitment protocols prevent study delays, reduce costs, and ensure data quality. Collaborating with community gatekeepers and establishing genuine partnerships is essential for accessing marginalized populations and building rapport with participants.
3. **Active and passive recruitment strategies**: The chapter explores both active (e.g., attending LGBT-friendly venues, reaching out to previous participants) and passive (e.g., posting flyers, online ads) recruitment strategies. Active recruitment builds visibility and trust, while passive methods reach a broader audience. Culturally sensitive materials and consistent engagement are key to making these strategies successful.
4. **Retention and study engagement strategies**: Retaining participants requires building respect and trust through regular communication, personalized interactions, and culturally sensitive practices. Study retention is enhanced by maintaining contact with participants, conducting studies in preferred venues, and offering appropriate incentives that reflect participants' time and effort.
5. **Forming culturally competent research teams**: Research teams should reflect the cultural and social dynamics of the community they are studying. Including Black gay researchers on study teams improves recruitment, data quality, and participant trust. Culturally congruent research leadership is critical for engaging Black SMM, as participants are more likely to trust researchers who share similar backgrounds and experiences.
6. **Distinguishing between community-based vs. community-placed research**: The chapter distinguishes between community-based research, which involves active collaboration with the community throughout the research process, and community-placed research, where the community serves as a setting for data collection without substantial involvement. True community-based research fosters trust and ensures that interventions are culturally relevant and sustainable.
7. **Ethical considerations for informed consent documents**: Ethical considerations, such as providing clear, transparent informed consent, are critical for building trust. Black SMM express concerns about data privacy and the adequacy of consent forms. Researchers should address these concerns by ensuring that consent forms are culturally sensitive, transparent, and demonstrate care for participants.

References

Cahill, S., Taylor, S. W., Elsesser, S. A., Mena, L., Hickson, D., & Mayer, K. H. (2017). Stigma, medical mistrust, and perceived racism may affect PrEP awareness and uptake in black compared to white gay and bisexual men in Jackson, Mississippi and Boston, Massachusetts. *AIDS Care, 29*(11), 1351–1358. https://doi.org/10.1080/09540121.2017.1300633

Calabrese, S. K., Kalwicz, D. A., Dovidio, J. F., Rao, S., Modrakovic, D. X., Boone, C. A., Magnus, M., Kharfen, M., Patel, V. V., & Zea, M. C. (2023). Targeted social marketing of PrEP and the stigmatization of Black sexual minority men. *PLoS One, 18*(5), e0285329. https://doi.org/10.1371/journal.pone.0285329

Dangerfield, D., II, & Wylie, C. (2022). Identifying ethical and culturally responsive research activities to build trust and improve participation of Black sexual minority men in pre-exposure prophylaxis telehealth clinical trials: Qualitative study. *JMIR Human Factors, 9*(1), e28798. https://doi.org/10.2196/28798

Dangerfield, D. T., II, Smith, L. R., Anderson, J. N., Bruce, O. J., Farley, J., & Bluthenthal, R. (2017). Sexual positioning practices and sexual risk among Black gay and bisexual men: A life course perspective. *AIDS and Behavior, 22*(6), 1919–1931. https://doi.org/10.1007/s10461-017-1948-6

Dangerfield, D. T., II, Harawa, N. T., McWells, C., Hilliard, C., & Bluthenthal, R. N. (2018). Exploring the preferences of a culturally congruent, peer-based HIV prevention intervention for black men who have sex with men. *Sexual Health, 15*(5), 424–430. https://doi.org/10.1071/SH18057

Dangerfield, D. T., II, Heidari, O., Cooper, J., Allen, S., & Lucas, G. M. (2020). Motivations for opioid and stimulant use among drug using black sexual minority men: A life course perspective. *Drug and Alcohol Dependence, 215*, 108224. https://doi.org/10.1016/j.drugalcdep.2020.108224

Dangerfield, D. T., II, Cooper, J., Heidari, O., Allen, S., Winder, T. J. A., & Lucas, G. M. (2021a). Nursing and health care preferences among opioid and stimulant using Black sexual minority men: An exploratory study. *Journal of the Association of Nurses in AIDS Care, 32*(5), e30–e39. https://doi.org/10.1097/JNC.0000000000000201

Dangerfield, D. T., II, Wylie, C., & Anderson, J. N. (2021b). Conducting virtual, synchronous focus groups among Black sexual minority men: Qualitative study. *JMIR Public Health and Surveillance, 7*(2), e22980. https://doi.org/10.2196/22980

Dangerfield, D. T., II, Anderson, J. N., Wylie, C., Arrington-Sanders, R., Bluthenthal, R. N., Beyrer, C., & Farley, J. E. (2022a). Refining a multicomponent intervention to increase perceived HIV risk and PrEP initiation: Focus group study among Black sexual minority men. *JMIR Formative Research, 6*(8), e34181. https://doi.org/10.2196/34181

Dangerfield, D. T., II, Ober, A. J., Li, M. J., Allen, S., & Bluthenthal, R. N. (2022b). HIV treatment adherence strategies among virally suppressed Black sexual minority men in Baltimore, Maryland, and Los Angeles, California: A theory-based qualitative study. *Journal of the Association of Nurses in AIDS Care, 33*(1), 54–62. https://doi.org/10.1097/JNC.0000000000000304

Fahey, O. B., Carr, D. J., Ocean, E. M., Nittas, V., Kane, C. P., Monti, P. M., & Wray, T. B. (2024). Black social media influencers engage higher percentages of Black gay and bisexual men in online outreach for HIV prevention research relative to paid ads. *DIGITAL HEALTH, 10*, 20552076241253758. https://doi.org/10.1177/20552076241253758

Funk, C. (2022, April 7). *Black Americans' views of and engagement with science*. Pew Research Center. https://www.pewresearch.org/science/2022/04/07/black-americans-views-of-and-engagement-with-science/

Happell, B. (2007). Focus groups in nursing research: An appropriate method or the latest fad? *Nurse Researcher (through 2013); London, 14*(2), 18–24.

Hoppe, T. A., Litovitz, A., Willis, K. A., Meseroll, R. A., Perkins, M. J., Hutchins, B. I., Davis, A. F., Lauer, M. S., Valantine, H. A., Anderson, J. M., & Santangelo, G. M. (2019). Topic choice contributes to the lower rate of NIH awards to African-American/Black scientists. *Science Advances, 5*(10), eaaw7238. https://doi.org/10.1126/sciadv.aaw7238

Israel, B. A., Schulz, A. J., Parker, E. A., & Becker, A. B. (1998). Review of community-based research: Assessing partnership approaches to improve public health. *Annual Review of Public Health, 19*(1), 173–202. https://doi.org/10.1146/annurev.publhealth.19.1.173

Israel, B. A., Coombe, C. M., Cheezum, R. R., Schulz, A. J., McGranaghan, R. J., Lichtenstein, R., Reyes, A. G., Clement, J., & Burris, A. (2010). Community-based participatory research: A capacity-building approach for policy advocacy aimed at eliminating health disparities. *American Journal of Public Health, 100*(11), 2094–2102. https://doi.org/10.2105/AJPH.2009.170506

Magnus, M., Franks, J., Griffith, S., Arnold, M. P., Goodman, K., Wheeler, D. P., & HPTN 061 Study Group. (2014). Engaging, recruiting, and retaining Black men who have sex with men in research studies: Don't underestimate the importance of staffing--lessons learned from HPTN 061, the BROTHERS study. *Journal of Public Health Management and Practice: JPHMP, 20*(6), E1–E9. https://doi.org/10.1097/PHH.0000000000000025

Pöyry, E., Reinikainen, H., & Luoma-Aho, V. (2022). The role of social media influencers in public health communication: Case COVID-19 pandemic. *International Journal of Strategic Communication, 16*(3), 469–484. https://doi.org/10.1080/1553118X.2022.2042694

Quinn, K., Dickson-Gomez, J., Zarwell, M., Pearson, B., & Lewis, M. (2018). "A gay man and a doctor are just like, a recipe for destruction": How racism and homonegativity in healthcare settings influence PrEP uptake among young Black MSM. *AIDS and Behavior, 23*, 1951–1963. https://doi.org/10.1007/s10461-018-2375-z

Scharff, D. P., Mathews, K. J., Jackson, P., Hoffsuemmer, J., Martin, E., & Edwards, D. (2010). More than Tuskegee: Understanding mistrust about research participation. *Journal of Health Care for the Poor and Underserved, 21*(3), 879–897. https://doi.org/10.1353/hpu.0.0323

Wei, C., McFarland, W., Colfax, G. N., Fuqua, V., & Raymond, H. F. (2012). Reaching Black men who have sex with men: A comparison between respondent-driven sampling and time-location sampling. *Sexually Transmitted Infections, 88*, 622–626. https://doi.org/10.1136/sextrans-2012-050619

White, J. J., Dangerfield, D. T., II, & Grieb, S. M. (2019). Methodological considerations for conducting focus groups in HIV prevention research among Black men who have sex with men. *Public Health Nursing, 36*(3), 439–445. https://doi.org/10.1111/phn.12592

Chapter 4
Using Person-Centered Statistical Approaches for Study and Intervention Design

Chapter Objectives

1. Describe the utility of person-centered versus variable centered analyses in sexual health prevention science among Black sexual minority men (SMM).
2. Review examples of person-centered analyses in minority sexual health prevention science.
3. Examine the role of person-centered approaches on intervention design for Black SMM.

The Role of Statistical Analyses in Sexual Health Prevention Science

Statistical methods use quantitative data, which is numerical and measured, to identify patterns, relationships, and trends between variables. These findings can be generalized across larger populations or datasets, allowing for predictions, inferences, and evidence-based decision-making in various fields such as science, business, and social research. Using statistical techniques enhances the depth of insights that can be derived from quantitative data. Specifically, statistics help prevention scientists (and other researchers) make inferences and predictions about a population based on a sample of data, evaluate and test theories or assumptions, and provide evidence for making informed decisions. Qualitative data, while rich and detailed, is more subjective and harder to generalize than statistics, which makes quantitative data a powerful tool for evidence-based decision-making, policy, and practice. Prevention scientists (and other researchers) can use quantitative data to make predictions about future events using statistics, which is key for generating effective

D. T. Dangerfield II, *Prevention Science & Targeted Methods for HIV/STI Research with Black Sexual Minority Men*,
https://doi.org/10.1007/978-3-031-85130-8_4

solutions for communities. Essentially, statistical analyses are fundamental for drawing valid and reliable conclusions and making informed public health decisions.

As discussed in Chaps. 1 and 2, the "risk" and "vulnerability" among Black SMM is contextual and varies within the population. Not everyone engages in the same behaviors and individual vulnerability to disease acquisition varies depending upon many different factors. Additionally, broad-brush health interventions may not be effective for everyone. Put simply, not everyone is the same. Therefore, prevention scientists, clinicians, and interventionists must understand the diverse needs of the community. Otherwise, general public health messages and programs will be largely ineffective. Uptake and adherence to effective treatment medications will also be low. For example, although data suggest that Black gay and bisexual men generally have a high acute HIV risk, only 52–65% of those who seroconverted had an indication for PrEP based on the CDC's guidelines (Ezennia et al., 2019; Hoots et al., 2016; Lancki et al., 2018). This suggests that the current indicators that clinicians use to identify and recommend PrEP might be insufficient or incomplete. It could also mean that there could be new, different, or emerging risk factors among this group that have not yet been identified.

Since Black SMM are not a homogeneous population that shares one undifferentiated profile of "risk", they can be characterized by subgroups that are comprised of uniquely different behaviors, attitudes, and experiences. Individuals who share similar characteristics could comprise distinct subgroups that differ in their behaviors, vulnerabilities, and their likelihood for prevention activities (such as PrEP use for HIV prevention). Hypothetically, those subgroups should be targeted differently using specific intervention approaches that address their unique differential vulnerabilities. However, intervention and treatment guidelines typically rely on variable-centered measures of behavioral risk (e.g., condom use, STI history, or relationship status). These measures inadequately identify the highest-risk individuals, as evidenced by data showing the relatively low prevalence of Black SMM who seroconverted based on those indicators (Hoots et al., 2016; Lancki et al., 2018). Given this, evaluating sexual health risk and vulnerability among Black SMM requires person-centered statistical approaches to identify the differential vulnerability among population subgroups, design targeted interventions, and identify best candidates for treatment recommendations.

Person-Centered Analysis

Person-centered statistical methods focus on identifying and understanding subgroups that share similar characteristics or experiences within a population (Howard & Hoffman, 2018; Vincent et al., 2019). Specifically, person-centered analyses identify and characterize profiles of individuals based on patterns of scores across multiple variables to identify subgroups within a dataset. In person-centered analyses, the goal is to identify meaningful and interpretable groups of individuals who share similar characteristics, profiles, or trajectories. Person-centered analyses are useful for exploring heterogeneity within a population, identifying distinct subgroups with different profiles or trajectories, and understanding how individuals within each subgroup differ in their responses or outcomes. Common person-centered statistical techniques include cluster analysis, latent class analysis (LCA), latent profile analysis (LPA), growth mixture modeling (GMM), and latent transition analysis (LTA). These methods are often used in psychology, sociology, and other social sciences and are also useful in prevention science.

For example, a hypothetical study might want to examine the sexual health behaviors and outcomes of LGBTQ+ youth. Researchers could conduct a cluster analysis to identify distinct subgroups within this population based on factors such as sexual orientation, gender identity, frequency of sexual activity, types of sexual partners, and access to sexual health resources. The analysis might identify one subgroup that consists of transgender youth who frequently engage in sexual activity but have limited access to gender-affirming healthcare and education, resulting in higher rates of STIs for them. Another subgroup could include bisexual youth who engage in both same-sex and opposite-sex relationships and report higher levels of psychological distress related to societal stigma, which might affect their STI outcomes differently than the trans youth. This person-centered approach highlights the diversity within the LGBTQ+ youth population, uncovering specific needs and risks that might be overlooked in a variable-centered analysis such as a logistic regression model. The findings from person-centered analyses can inform targeted sexual health interventions for population subgroups to improve inclusive healthcare services by addressing the unique needs, behaviors, and risk factors of each subgroup. Person-centered statistical methods are particularly valuable in sexual minority prevention science because they allow researchers to identify and understand diverse subgroups within the population, including the complexity of the combined experiences regarding race, sexuality, adversity, and marginalization. Person-centered statistics inform policymakers about the specific needs and challenges of different subgroups, leading to more informed and equitable policy decisions. Targeting subgroups for prevention and treatment activities is more effective and economical than trying to intervene on everyone in the population. Additionally, my research using mixture models shows that only small proportions of SMM samples have high-risk profiles that require intervention relative to others in the sample (Dangerfield II et al., 2018a, b). This suggests that prevention activities could target a small population of highest risk SMM instead of general samples.

Person-Centered Versus Variable-Centered Analyses

Variable-centered approaches, such as correlation analysis and regression analysis, focus on examining relationships between the variables within a dataset, typically with the goal of identifying associations or testing the hypotheses of theoretical constructs. Variable-centered analyses are useful for exploring patterns of association between variables, testing hypotheses about causal relationships, and identifying underlying dimensions or constructs that explain variability in the data. These analyses often assume that relationships between variables are uniform across the entire population, potentially overlooking unique experiences and needs of population subgroups, especially in minority communities. The focus in these types of analyses is to understand the relationships between variables themselves rather than group individuals based on their scores on those variables. For example, a regression analysis for a variable-centered approach typically aims to understand the relationship between a dependent variable and one or more independent variables, focusing on how changes in predictor variables influence the outcome variable.

Consider a hypothetical study examining the impact of drug use and age on syphilis incidence among Black gay men. Using data from 500 patients, the analysis might involve fitting a multiple regression model in which syphilis incidence is the dependent variable and drug use and age rates are the independent variables. The results could reveal that both drug use and age significantly predict syphilis incidence, showing that drug use has a stronger effect. This variable-centered analysis would help prevention scientists understand the importance of demographic and behavioral factors on STI outcomes and potentially inform interventions. However, variable-centered approaches may fail to account for nuanced cultural, social, and economic contexts that significantly influence health outcomes in minority populations and create vulnerable subgroups. Therefore, person-centered analysis focuses on grouping individuals based on similarities in their profiles or trajectories, whereas variable-centered analysis focuses on relationships between variables. In person-centered analysis, the unit of analysis is the individual or case, whereas in variable-centered analysis, the unit of analysis is the variable or item. Person-centered analyses identify meaningful subgroups of individuals with distinct characteristics or outcomes, whereas variable-centered analysis aims to understand patterns of association or underlying structures among variables. Person-centered statistics also help identify and validate the varied lived experiences of Black SMM and fosters a more inclusive and nuanced understanding of their vulnerabilities, needs, and strengths.

Mixture Modeling for Person Centered Analyses

Mixture models such as LCA, LPA, and LTA are person-centered approaches that can help researchers obtain a more holistic picture of population subgroups including their profiles or typologies and foreshadow their membership in a unique subgroup longitudinally (Lanza et al., 2010; Muthen, 2004). Mixture models assume that the population is comprised of discrete subgroups or unique "typologies." The concept of typologies (or subgroups) comes from taxometric studies in which diagnoses in psychopathology research could be distinctly characterized by a collection of symptoms (Meehl, 1992, 1995). For example, the collection of factors that comprise a depression diagnosis is very different from those of anxiety or a psychotic disorder. The same notion of a "typology" with distinctive features could be considered for Black SMM regarding their risk behaviors, vulnerabilities, or motivations to change behaviors. From a prevention science and public health perspective, it is essential to identify factors that make a particular typology distinctive because these unique features are what contribute to differential vulnerability among population subgroups. The differences that mixture modeling can identify can also indicate the elements that are needed for targeted interventions to address the features that make the people in the typology uniquely vulnerable. Latent statuses can represent unobservable subgroups within a population and provide crucial insights into the progression of health-related behaviors, conditions, or attitudes. Research on unique typologies among Black SMM have been insightful but is still in the preliminary stages and mostly limited to HIV research (Dangerfield II et al., 2018b; Scheidell et al., 2021; Turpin et al., 2020). Still, the advantage of mixture models is that they offer a flexible approach than can handle complex data and provide detailed information about the nature of each profile to identifying subgroups without requiring prior assumptions about the details or number of groups.

Latent Profile Analysis

LPA is probabilistic model-based strategy that identifies the profiles of subgroups within a population based on continuous variables (Nylund et al., 2007). A 1-profile model suggests a single undifferentiated population, whereas multiple profiles (e.g., 3 or 4) suggest there are hidden "mixtures" (or subgroups) within the population that have a unique composition of attitudes, behaviors, or experiences. Two factors are considered in determining the unique features of a LPA profile (Morin et al., 2016). The first is the absolute level of an indicator (intercept) and the extent to which the indicator is above or below average levels for the entire group. The second factor is the "shape" of the profile when all indicators are examined as a whole. This considers what the profile looks like when all of the indicators are viewed together in the form of a plot. This information is useful in characterizing members of a particular profile and emphasizing what distinguishes membership in one profile from another. For example, a 3-profile solution can identify one group that has high scores on all facets of health behaviors, another group can have lower scores on all of the indicators, and a third can have a mixed profile that has some health behavior scores above and some below the average of the group. These distinctions in level and shape give a profile its unique characterization and nomenclature.

Figure 4.1 provides a graphic of a hypothetical 3-profile LPA solution on a study to identify measures of STI risk perceptions among Black SMM. One latent "risk perception profile" could involve a subgroup of men with relatively high mean levels of perceived susceptibility, severity and benefits, but relatively low scores for perceived barriers, average scores for cues to action and high scores for likelihood of action, efficacy and locus of control (the black line). A second profile (the orange line) is average with respect to HBM-related constructs as well as cues to action, likelihood of action, self-efficacy and locus of control expectancies. The third

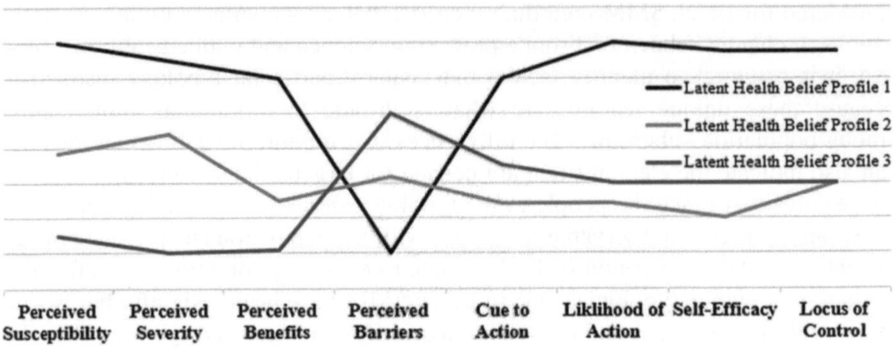

Fig. 4.1 Hypothetical LPA solution guided by HBM-related constructs

profile (blue line) has very low scores on susceptibility, severity and benefits, much higher scores on barriers, and average scores for the remaining measures of cues to action, likelihood of action, self-efficacy, and locus of control. These groups have different health beliefs, process information differently, and are therefore differentially vulnerable for STIs. From a prevention standpoint, these different profiles require targeted interventions to address their distinct vulnerability, which cannot be identified using variable-centered approaches (e.g., regression, correlation, or factor loadings) because a single set of parameters is obtained for the whole population.

Latent Class Analysis

LCA is another form of mixture modeling that is useful method to identify how a set of categorical indicators create different profiles of risk (Lanza & Rhoades, 2011) although continuous variables can also be included in models with categorical variables. Similar to LPA, LCA quantifies both the profiles of co-occurring indicators such as behaviors, attitudes, and/or experiences and identifies the means (for continuous variables) and conditional probabilities (for categorical variables) of those factors within latent classes (Lanza & Rhoades, 2011; Muthen, 2004). In LPA, all of the indicators are continuous variables.

I have published several studies using LCA showing that Black SMM and other minority groups can be characterized by multiple subgroups with distinct profiles of vulnerability (Dangerfield II et al., 2018a, 2018b, 2021; Turpin et al., 2020). For example, we used data from the HIV Prevention Trials Network (HPTN) 073 study to use the categorical indicators of CDC PrEP screening guidelines (i.e., relationship status, condom use, number of sexual partners, substance use, STI history, and partner HIV status) among a sample of ~225 HIV-negative Black SMM in the U.S. (Dangerfield II et al., 2021). The LCA in that study identified three distinct profiles of HIV risk behaviors and essentially differential vulnerability in the sample: (1) "Single with Condomless Partners" who comprised 69% of the sample, (2) "Single with Multiple Partners" comprising 19% of the sample, and (3) "Serodiscordant Partners" (12% of the sample) (Table 4.1).

The conditional probabilities for individuals classified as Single with Multiple Partners were the highest for having greater than three male partners, substance use before sex, and receiving an STI diagnosis. Serodiscordant Partners had a 100% conditional probability of condomless sex and having a male partner living with HIV. Additionally, Black SMM who initiated PrEP were almost 40% less likely to be classified as Single with Condomless Partners than Serodiscordant Partners compared to those who did not inditiate PrEP (Dangerfield II et al., 2021). This analysis added to the knowledge of how sexual risk profiles are associated with PrEP use along with a more accurate HIV risk assessment for Black SMM that is not currently available to interventionists and clinical providers. These findings supported hypotheses and data suggesting that CDC guidelines may be too general and inaccurately identify Black SMM at greatest risk for HIV. These data also highlights the need for more tailored guidelines and interventions that consider the specific risk profiles and behaviors within this community, ensuring that those at the highest risk are accurately identified and receive appropriate prevention resources.

Table 4.1 Latent class distribution of sexual risk indicators (n = 226)

Latent Class Indicators	Class 1: Single with Condomless Partners 157 (69.4%)	Class 2: Single with Multiple Partners 43 (19.0%)	Class 3: Serodiscordant Partners 26 (11.5%)
Relationship status			
Single or not in a committed relationship	0.841	0.996	0.467
Relationship	0.159	0.034	0.533
Condomless IAI or RAI	0.862	0.905	1.00
≥3 male partners	0.313	0.936	0.190
Substance use before sex	0.574	0.581	0.571
STI history	0.082	0.426	0.000
Any HIV positive male partners	0.000	0.466	1.00

Latent Transition Analysis

The attitudes, behaviors, circumstances, and disease vulnerabilities of communities can change over time. LTA is a longitudinal analysis that examines the likelihood of changes in those conditions or vulnerabilities over time (Lanza et al., 2010). LTA extends LCA by adding a longitudinal dimension the study of subgroups within a population. While LCA and LPA classify subgroups at a one time-point, LTA goes a step further by analyzing how individuals transition between those latent classes over multiple time points. This extension allows prevention scientists to better understand the dynamics and changes of behavior or disease vulnerability. Analytically, follow-up analyses in a 1-year study with baseline (T_1), 6-month (T_2), and 12-month (T_3) follow-up can be used to determine "who" is moving between status profiles for example. First, latent status membership is estimated at each time point, which yields estimates of profile intercepts and profile sizes. Then, the model estimates indicate the likelihood of the subgroups moving or changing profile membership between time points, which includes the likelihood of profile status at T_3 conditioned on prior profile membership at T_2 and also T_2 conditioned on T_1. In some cases, individuals might remain in their particular status while in other situations they may shift to a different profile characterized by less "risk." By identifying and modeling these transitions, LTA allows researchers to understand how individuals move between different health states or behavioral patterns, such as stages of substance use, or adherence to treatment protocols. LTA is particularly valuable for evaluating the effectiveness of public health interventions, as it can reveal how specific strategies influence the probability of transitioning from a less desirable to a more desirable health status. Moreover, LTA can account for measurement error and accommodate complex longitudinal data, making it a powerful tool for capturing the dynamic nature of health behaviors and outcomes (Lanza et al., 2010).

We conducted an LTA to identify changes in sexual health vulnerability regarding racism, homophobia, and behavioral health indicators among ~1000 Black SMM in HPTN 061 (Turpin et al., 2020). Theoretically, we hypothesized that there would be distinct profiles of vulnerability and that over time they would change. The LTA model produced four initial subgroups: a "low-risk" status characterized by the lowest proportions of scores on the indicators and 3 "high-risk" statuses characterized by higher proportions on the score. All three high-risk statuses were associated with higher substance use than the low-risk status, with the greatest association observed with "high-risk status. Among participants above the median social support index, we observed greater percentages of maintenance of low-risk status (84.2% compared to 75.9%) and transition from high-risk to low-risk (63.5% compared to 44.6%) than those below or at the median social support index. Black SMM with above-average social support had better outcomes. Additionally, 63.5% moved from high-risk to low-risk, compared to 44.6% with lower support. Regression analysis showed that higher social support significantly reduced the risk of moving from low-risk to high-risk. Overall, LTA enhances the ability of prevention scientists to design targeted interventions and policies to improve community/population health.

Designing a Person-Centered Study

Consider an HIV/STI prevention study that examines how cognitive factors involving health beliefs, self-efficacy, and control expectancies could create subgroups with distinct vulnerabilities and behavioral outcomes among Black SMM. Hypothetically, some Black SMM might change from a profile with lower risk perceptions to one of higher risk perceptions over the course of their lives. Major life events, circumstances, or experiences may change the way they perceive the severity of disease or vulnerability to infection (Dangerfield II et al. 2017, 2020), but we don't know how people within the community might differ on these factors even though they belong to the same target group overall. Figure 4.2 provides a conceptual model that depicts how the role of time can be used with mixture modeling for a person-centered approach that examines this change. The first step would examine whether there are qualitatively distinct subgroups of Black SMM with unique profiles of vulnerability regarding levels of risk perceptions. The blue boxes represent the indicators that will be used to explore latent risk perception profiles. Since the indicators would be continuous (because individuals would provide responses to survey measures that involve scales or scores), LPA would be used to identify distinct subgroups (Fig. 4.2, Aim 1). Statistically, the unobserved latent profile (the orange circles with arrows pointing to the observed indicators in the blue boxes) causes the indicators to form a distinctive profile based on the pattern of item means. As an extension of that goal, the study could examine whether certain demographic, personal, and/or contextual factors help to characterize subgroup

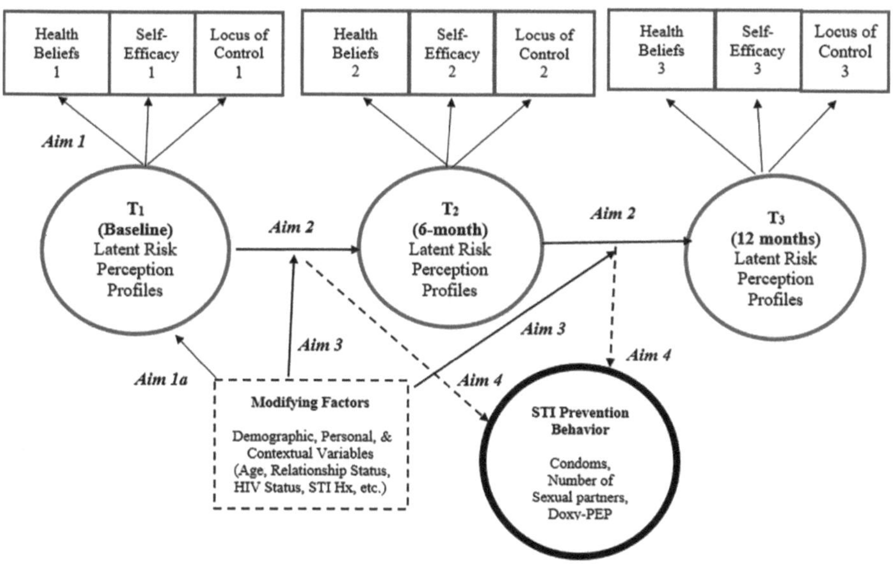

Fig. 4.2 Conceptual model of theoretically guided, longitudinal person centered analysis

membership (Fig. 4.2, Aim 1a). This involves covariate adjustments to the LPA model. A second Aim can examine whether membership in the unique profiles remains stable or changes over time (Fig. 4.2, Aim 2). This would be done using LTA to obtain probability estimates for the transitions across time (T_1 to T_2 and T_2 to T_3). This movement over time will be reflected in the transition probabilities (and can involve movement from high to low risk as well).

Related to this goal, the study can then examine the influence of specific demographic, personal, and contextual factors on change in risk status over time (Aim 3). This analysis examines whether certain factors prompt or instigate movement between statuses, for instance, whether STI test results have an influence on risk status. Then, analyses could examine relationships between risk profile membership (and change in risk profile status) and STI prevention behaviors including condom use, number of sexual partners, and STI post-exposure prophylaxis (Aim 4). Figure X depicts this part of the statistical modeling using stippled lines from the transition probabilities capturing change in status from T_1-T_2 and likewise from T_2-T_3 to the distal outcome (*STI Prevention Behavior*). Essentially, this portion of the model asks whether movement between status groups (i.e., lower to higher risk) is associated with greater engagement in health-compromising behaviors, demographic, personal or contextual factors. Identifying specific subgroups enables the design of targeted interventions that are more likely to effectively prevent STIs for particular segments of the population of Black SMM.

Conclusions

Person-centered analysis and variable-centered analysis represent different approaches to analyzing data, each with its own strengths and applications. The choice between the two approaches depends on the research questions, the nature of the data, and the goals of the analysis. However, person-centered statistical approaches are particularly useful when researchers are interested in exploring the diversity within a population and understanding how different subgroups might have unique characteristics or experiences. Person-centered statistics provide a more nuanced and detailed understanding of populations by recognizing and modeling individual and subgroup differences. The results of these types of analyses lead to more effective interventions, improved predictive accuracy, and better-informed policy decisions, ultimately enhancing the quality and impact of prevention science and practice. To effectively promote minority health, it is essential to complement variable-centered analyses with person-centered and mixed-methods approaches that capture the complexity and diversity of health determinants in these populations.

Raised Questions

1. What are the best indicators needed to identify the differences in sexual health vulnerability among Black SMM?
2. What are the practical applications of understanding individual differences in the context of the findings?
3. What kinds of interventions or policies can be designed from person-centered analyses?

Chapter Summary

This chapter explored the importance and utility of person-centered statistical approaches in sexual health prevention science, particularly among Black SMM. The chapter began by contrasting person-centered analyses with traditional variable-centered methods, emphasizing that while variable-centered approaches are useful for identifying relationships between variables across a population, they often overlook the heterogeneity within subgroups. Person-centered methods, such as latent class analysis (LCA) and latent profile analysis (LPA), are introduced as useful tools for identifying and characterizing distinct subgroups within a population based on shared behaviors, attitudes, and experiences. The chapter highlighted the limitations of current intervention and treatment guidelines, which often rely on broad, variable-centered measures of behavioral risk. These approaches can inadequately identify individuals at the highest risk for HIV and other STIs among Black SMM. In contrast, person-centered approaches allow for a more nuanced understanding of individual differences, enabling researchers to identify specific subgroups that might require tailored/targeted interventions. Examples of person-centered analyses in minority sexual health research were provided, illustrating how these methods can reveal the diversity within populations and inform the design of targeted, effective interventions. The chapter discussed the application of mixture models, including LPA, LCA, and latent transition analysis (LTA), to uncover unique typologies within Black SMM and track changes in risk profiles over time. These models help prevention scientists identify the factors that contribute to differential vulnerability and design interventions that are better suited to the specific needs of each subgroup. The chapter concluded by raising critical questions about the practical applications of person-centered analyses and their potential to inform policy and intervention design, advocating for the integration of person-centered approaches with variable-centered analyses to capture the complexity and diversity of health determinants in minority populations such as Black SMM.

Key Points

1. **Person-centered vs. variable-centered approaches**: Person-centered approaches identify distinct subgroups based on shared characteristics, while variable centered approaches identify the relationships between variables. This distinction is essential for identifying and addressing the diverse needs of Black SMM.
2. **The limitations of current HIV/STI prevention guidelines**: Current intervention guidelines for HIV and STI prevention often rely on general, variable-centered measures of risk, which may not adequately capture the diversity of behaviors and vulnerabilities among Black SMM. These guidelines can overlook high-risk individuals and subgroups, leading to less effective interventions.
3. **Mixture models to identify typologies**: Mixture models like LPA and LCA help prevention scientists identify unique typologies within Black SMM populations based on behaviors, attitudes, and experiences. These models reveal distinct profiles or subgroups that have different levels of vulnerability, allowing for more nuanced and personalized intervention strategies. LTA extends the analysis of subgroups by examining how individuals transition between different profiles over time.
4. **Targeted interventions**: The chapter emphasizes that person-centered approaches are essential for designing interventions for specific subgroups within a population. By identifying and understanding the unique characteristics of these subgroups, prevention scientists can create more effective, targeted interventions that address the specific vulnerabilities of each group.
5. **Applications to policy and practice**: Integrating person-centered analyses with variable-centered approaches in public health research provides a more comprehensive understanding of health determinants in minority populations, leading to more informed policy decisions and more equitable, impactful interventions for Black SMM.

References

Dangerfield, D. T., II, Carmack, C. C., Gilreath, T. D., & Duncan, D. T. (2018a). Latent classes of sexual positioning practices and sexual risk among men who have sex with men in Paris, France. *AIDS and Behavior, 22*(12), 4001–4008. https://doi.org/10.1007/s10461-018-2267-2

Dangerfield, D. T., II, Harawa, N. T., Smith, L. R., Jeffries, W. L., Baezconde-Garbanati, L., & Bluthenthal, R. (2018b). Latent classes of sexual risk among Black men who have sex with men and women. *Archives of Sexual Behavior, 47*(7), 2071–2080. https://doi.org/10.1007/s10508-017-1142-y

Dangerfield, D. T., II, Heidari, O., Cooper, J., Allen, S., & Lucas, G. M. (2020). Motivations for opioid and stimulant use among drug using black sexual minority men: A life course perspective. *Drug and Alcohol Dependence, 215*, 108224. https://doi.org/10.1016/j.drugalcdep.2020.108224

Dangerfield, D. T., II, Kuo, I., Magnus, M., Beauchamp, G., Fields, S. D., Nelson, L., Shoptaw, S., Wilton, L., & Wheeler, D. P. (2021). Sexual risk profiles among Black sexual minority men:

Implications for targeted PrEP messaging. *Archives of Sexual Behavior, 50*(7), 2947–2954. https://doi.org/10.1007/s10508-021-02066-w
Dangerfield, D. T., II, Smith, L. R., Anderson, J. N., Bruce, O. J., Farley, J., & Bluthenthal, R. (2017). Sexual positioning practices and sexual risk among Black gay and bisexual men: A life course perspective. *AIDS and Behavior, 22*(6), 1919–1931. https://doi.org/10.1007/s10461-017-1948-6
Ezennia, O., Geter, A., & Smith, D. K. (2019). The PrEP care continuum and Black men who have sex with men: A scoping review of published data on awareness, uptake, adherence, and retention in PrEP care. *AIDS and Behavior, 23*(10), 2654–2673. https://doi.org/10.1007/s10461-019-02641-2
Hoots, B. E., Finlayson, T., Nerlander, L., Paz-Bailey, G., Wortley, P., Todd, J., Sato, K., Flynn, C., German, D., Fukuda, D., Doherty, R., Wittke, C., Prachand, N., Benbow, N., Jimenez, A. D., Poe, J., Sheu, S., Novoa, A., Al-Tayyib, A., Xia, M., et al. (2016). Willingness to take, use of, and indications for pre-exposure prophylaxis among men who have sex with men—20 US cities, 2014. *Clinical Infectious Diseases, 63*(5), 672–677. https://doi.org/10.1093/cid/ciw367
Howard, M. C., & Hoffman, M. E. (2018). Variable-centered, person-centered, and person-specific approaches: Where theory meets the method. *Organizational Research Methods, 21*(4), 846–876. https://doi.org/10.1177/1094428117744021
Lancki, N., Almirol, E., Alon, L., McNulty, M., & Schneider, J. A. (2018). Preexposure prophylaxis guidelines have low sensitivity for identifying seroconverters in a sample of young Black MSM in Chicago. *AIDS, 32*(3), 383–392. https://doi.org/10.1097/QAD.0000000000001710
Lanza, S. T., Patrick, M. E., & Maggs, J. L. (2010). Latent transition analysis: Benefits of a latent variable approach to modeling transitions in substance use. *Journal of Drug Issues, 40*(1), 93–120.
Lanza, S. T., & Rhoades, B. L. (2011). Latent class analysis: An alternative perspective on subgroup analysis in prevention and treatment. *Prevention Science, 14*(2), 157–168. https://doi.org/10.1007/s11121-011-0201-1
Meehl, P. E. (1992). Factors and taxa, traits and types, differences of degree and differences in kind. *Journal of Personality, 60*(1), 117–174. https://doi.org/10.1111/j.1467-6494.1992.tb00269.x
Meehl, P. E. (1995). Bootstraps taxometrics: Solving the classification problem in psychopathology. *American Psychologist, 50*(4), 266–275. https://doi.org/10.1037/0003-066X.50.4.266
Morin, A. J. S., Boudrias, J.-S., Marsh, H. W., Madore, I., & Desrumaux, P. (2016). Further reflections on disentangling shape and level effects in person-centered analyses: An illustration exploring the dimensionality of psychological health. *Structural Equation Modeling: A Multidisciplinary Journal, 23*, 438–454. https://doi.org/10.1080/10705511.2015.1116077
Muthen, B. (2004). Latent variable analysis. In *The sage handbook of quantitative methodology for the social sciences* (pp. 345–368). Sage.
Nylund, K. L., Asparouhov, T., & Muthén, B. O. (2007). Deciding on the number of classes in latent class analysis and growth mixture modeling: A Monte Carlo simulation study. *Structural Equation Modeling: A Multidisciplinary Journal, 14*(4), 535–569. https://doi.org/10.1080/10705510701575396
Scheidell, J. D., Dyer, T. V., Hucks-Ortiz, C., Abrams, J., Mazumdar, M., Cleland, C., Irvine, N., Turpin, R. E., Severe, M., Mayer, K., & Khan, M. (2021). Characterisation of social support following incarceration among black sexual minority men and transgender women in the HPTN 061 cohort study. *BMJ Open, 11*(9), e053334. https://doi.org/10.1136/bmjopen-2021-053334
Turpin, R. E., Dyer, T. V., Dangerfield, D. T., Liu, H., & Mayer, K. H. (2020). Syndemic latent transition analysis in the HPTN 061 cohort: Prospective interactions between trauma, mental health, social support, and substance use. *Drug and Alcohol Dependence, 214*, 108106. https://doi.org/10.1016/j.drugalcdep.2020.108106
Vincent, W., Peterson, J. L., Storholm, E. D., Huebner, D. M., Neilands, T. B., Calabrese, S. K., Rebchook, G. M., Tan, J. Y., Pollack, L., & Kegeles, S. M. (2019). A person-centered approach to HIV-related protective and risk factors for young Black men who have sex with men: Implications for pre-exposure prophylaxis and HIV treatment as prevention. *AIDS and Behavior, 23*(10), 2803–2815. https://doi.org/10.1007/s10461-019-02630-5

Chapter 5
Contemporary and Culturally Responsive Considerations for Qualitative Methods

Chapter Objectives

1. Identify the value qualitative methodology in sexual health prevention science.
2. Describe contemporary qualitative methodologies for research with Black sexual minority men (SMM).
3. Enhance cultural competency and ethical conduct in qualitative research with Black SMM.

The Value of Qualitative Methodology in HIV/STI Prevention Science

Qualitative studies are useful for gathering personal, detailed, and contextual data on topics about which little is known (Gill et al., 2008). Unlike quantitative methods (discussed in Chap. 4), qualitative research allows prevention scientists to explore complex social dynamics and personal narratives that are often overlooked with detail and nuance (Creswell & Poth, 2016; DiCicco-Bloom & Crabtree, 2006). Qualitative methodology plays a crucial role in HIV/STI prevention science by providing in-depth and nuanced insights into the behaviors, attitudes, and social contexts of disparate and marginalized communities such as Black SMM in ways that quantitative methods might overlook (Wilson et al., 2016). The insights gained from qualitative research are essential for sexual health intervention design (and implementation) because they allow and encourage people to discuss issues they might not be able to disclose in quantitative surveys, leading to rich, detailed data and a deeper understanding of the factors that increase risk and vulnerability (Wilson et al., 2016).

D. T. Dangerfield II, *Prevention Science & Targeted Methods for HIV/STI Research with Black Sexual Minority Men*,
https://doi.org/10.1007/978-3-031-85130-8_5

Using key qualitative methods such as in-depth interviews, focus groups, and ethnography, scientists can examine the experiences of individuals to better understand the reasons behind sexual health behaviors (Creswell & Poth, 2016). Through detailed discussions and observations, researchers have uncovered important reasons for uptake of prevention interventions (or lack thereof), including condom use, HIV testing, and PrEP (Arnold et al., 2014; Quinn et al., 2018, 2019). Prevention scientists can then design interventions that are more relevant and acceptable to the community by understanding the specific needs, preferences, and cultural contexts of subpopulations (von Hippel, 2018; Wilson et al., 2016). Qualitative studies have informed the design, implementation, and dissemination of effective interventions by providing contextual perspectives of HIV/STI vulnerability, including the influence of cultural and social norms. This user-centered (or person-centered, see Chap. 4) approach to intervention design enhances the effectiveness of interventions by ensuring they are appropriate for the intended community and address the unique facilitators and barriers within community contexts (von Hippel, 2018; Wilson et al., 2016). Qualitative methods can also identify the characteristics of protective health factors such as peer support, resourceful neighborhoods, and the qualities of preferred clinicians (Dangerfield II et al., 2018, 2021a; 2022b).

My research has utilized qualitative approaches to identify nuanced understandings of sexuality, behavioral health, and community needs among Black gay and bisexual men. I have personally conducted more than 200 in-depth interviews, 50 focus groups, and 400 hours of observations in clinical and community settings, gathering crucial contextual information regarding factors such as preferred health communication approaches (Dangerfield II et al., 2022a), key influencers (Dangerfield II et al., 2018), and cultural barriers to intervention uptake (Dangerfield II et al., 2022a). Participants in my studies generally mention that they share information with me that they have not or will not share with others partly due to assumptions about my in-group membership and beliefs that others will not understand or "care" about their experiences (Dangerfield II et al., 2021b, 2022a, b; White et al., 2019). These types of sentiments suggest that optimal qualitative research conduct among Black SMM could be prohibited because research mistrust remains prevalent. Other cross-cultural studies have found similar challenges in which historical injustices and cultural differences have led to deep-seated skepticism and reluctance to participate in research, ultimately impacting the quality and accuracy of data collected (Liamputtong, 2010). Typical study designs, teams, and approaches might affect the quality of qualitative data collection and analysis among Black SMM because they often fail to adequately account for cultural nuances, historical trauma, or their social experiences. This oversight can lead to a lack of trust, reduced participant engagement, and potential biases in the data (Liamputtong, 2010). Therefore, qualitative methodology in HIV/STI prevention science must be refined to obtain high quality data and conduct ethical research with Black SMM (White et al., 2019). This chapter offers advanced considerations for conducting in-depth interviews, focus groups, and ethnographic research within contemporary qualitative methodologies in HIV/STI prevention science among Black SMM, drawing upon insights from my research to enhance data collection and analysis and maximize targeted prevention science and methodology for this population.

In-Depth Interviews

In-depth interviews involve a researcher asking detailed questions about the experiences, attitudes, beliefs, or behaviors of one participant at a time (Gill et al., 2008). In-depth interviews are a useful method to consider when there is highly sensitive information involved such as experiences of adversity, trauma, or HIV/STIs diagnoses. In-depth interviews can yield higher quality data than other qualitative methods such as focus groups because participants may not completely discuss sensitive issues in a group setting (Guest et al., 2017; Johnstone, 2017). Since sexual health involves sensitive topics that often involve stigma, shame, and potentially illicit behaviors (e.g., sex work, drug use), in-depth interviews can provide a safer opportunity for people to share their experiences and perspectives with researchers than a focus group or survey questionnaire. For some Black SMM, the in-depth interview would be a better choice for research participation than a focus group or a clinical trial because some may have never shared some of their experiences regarding trauma or sexuality with others and they may disclose more information to researchers in a one-on-one interview than a focus group. Depending upon the topic, an in-depth interview is the only context in which some individuals will (and maybe should) discuss sensitive personal information, especially because sexuality, substance use, and mental health is still taboo in some communities. Moreover, the interpersonal dynamics between the researcher and participant impacts data collection, analysis, and findings (DiCicco-Bloom & Crabtree, 2006) in ways that are underdiscussed in HIV/STI prevention science. Therefore, researchers must be intentional regarding this methodology when selecting and training interviewers and conducting in-depth interviews for prevention research with Black SMM.

Considerations for In-Depth Interviewers in HIV/STI Prevention Science with Black Sexual Minority Men

The interviewer is essential in shaping the data collection and analysis in in-depth interviews. The interviewer is responsible for establishing rapport and trust, asking sensitive questions in nimble ways, managing potential emotional upset from participants, and interpreting the conversation correctly (della Porta, 2014). Participants may be more likely to share detailed, honest, and sensitive information when they feel comfortable and trust the interviewer (Song & Parker, 1995). The interviewer must also be sensitive and familiar enough with the cultural context to obtain and understand a wide range of truthful and detailed responses (Kanuha, 2000). Therefore, the characteristics, skills, demeanor, and approach of the interviewer substantially shapes the quality, depth, and validity of the data collected (della Porta, 2014; DiCicco-Bloom & Crabtree, 2006; Kanuha, 2000). Having a culturally similar interviewer can further enhance the benefits of qualitative methodology by fostering a deeper sense of understanding and connection, leading to more authentic and comprehensive insights with Black SMM (Kanuha, 2000).

Having a culturally similar interviewer in qualitative research offers numerous advantages that enhance the overall quality of the data collection and analysis. First, culturally similar interviewers can establish rapport and trust quickly because participants feel more comfortable and understood by someone who shares their cultural background, leading to richer, more detailed responses (Dunbar et al., 2002; Kanuha, 2000). Additionally, culturally similar interviewers can better interpret subtle nuances, idioms, and non-verbal responses that are specific to the participant's culture, which ensures a more accurate understanding of their responses and more relevant interview probes (Dunbar et al., 2002; Kanuha, 2000). Culturally similar interviewers are also more understanding of cultural sensitivities that may make participants more comfortable, which helps to frame questions in respectful and appropriate ways (Croot et al., 2011; Jandt, 2017). Having study team members who established a rapport with Black SMM has been a key component of successful recruitment and qualitative data collection in my work (See Chap. 3). Overall, these factors contribute to a more holistic representation of the participants' perspectives, ultimately enhancing the meaning of the research findings (Creswell & Poth, 2016).

Black SMM often express a preference for data collection to be conducted by individuals who are either Black, gay, or both (Dangerfield II et al., 2018, 2021a, 2022a). This preference is rooted in the belief that these researchers are more likely to be trustworthy and possess a deeper understanding of the cultural context and lived experiences unique to Black SMM. Participants feel that researchers who share their racial and/or sexual identity are more empathetic to the challenges they face, which can foster a sense of comfort and openness during the data collection process. This trust is crucial for obtaining accurate, honest, and comprehensive data, as participants may be more willing to disclose sensitive information to someone they perceive as having a shared background and a genuine investment in their community's well-being (Dangerfield II et al., 2021a; Dangerfield II & Wylie, 2022). Moreover, the presence of culturally similar researchers can help to mitigate feelings of exploitation or mistrust that have historically been associated with research in marginalized communities (Dangerfield II et al., 2022a; Dangerfield II & Wylie, 2022), thereby enhancing the overall quality of the research findings. More work is needed to better understand the elements of cultural similarities and difference that affect data collection and analysis in HIV/STI prevention science among Black SMM. Understanding these elements will be key to developing more effective, culturally responsive research methodologies that not only improve data accuracy but also foster greater trust and engagement from Black SMM.

When a culturally different interviewer conducts qualitative research, it is essential minimize cultural barriers and enhance data quality (Liamputtong, 2010). This can be achieved through strategies such as cultural sensitivity training, employing intercultural communication skills, and involving local collaborators to ensure that the research findings are more accurately reflective of the participants' true perspectives. Moreover, incorporating a reflective approach, where interviewers continuously assess and adjust their methods based on participants' feedback, ensures a more responsive and respectful research process (Jootun et al., 2009). Establishing trust with participants is crucial, and this can be facilitated by demonstrating genuine interest in and respect for their cultural backgrounds (Dangerfield II et al., 2021a; Dangerfield II & Wylie, 2022). Additionally, using language and terminology that resonates with the participants' experiences, and seeking guidance from cultural insiders or community leaders, can further bridge the cultural gap. By implementing these strategies, researchers can not only improve the authenticity and depth of the data collected but also foster a research environment where participants feel valued and understood, ultimately leading to richer and more meaningful insights.

Overall, the interviewer's competence and approach directly affect the richness, reliability, and validity of the qualitative data collected. Establishing rapport and trust with participants is essential because it encourages open and honest sharing of information for optimal data collection and analysis (Creswell & Poth, 2016; Dickson-Swift et al., 2007; Liamputtong, 2010). Additionally, the interviewer's own biases, beliefs, and attitudes can unconsciously influence how questions are asked and how responses are interpreted (Jootun et al., 2009). An interviewer's body language, tone of voice, and facial expressions can affect how participants respond potentially affecting the authenticity of the data (Johnson & Rowlands, 2012). The interviewer's understanding of the research context and the participant's background allows for more nuanced and relevant questioning (DiCicco-Bloom & Crabtree, 2006), which can lead to more meaningful and contextually rich data. They must be able to probe deeply without leading or emotionally triggering the participants, ensuring that the responses are genuine and reflective of the participants' true thoughts and feelings.

Managing Participant Upset from Disclosing Traumatic Experiences

Some Black SMM disclose and describe horrific stories about painful past histories of violence, abuse, and despair during in-depth interviews. Between 30% and 40% of Black gay men in my studies have disclosed experiences of childhood sexual abuse in in-depth interviews (Dangerfield II et al., 2017, 2020), which occasionally leads derails the conversation from the research topic as they reflect on the past when they had limited support as gay-identified men experiencing childhood trauma. Some Black gay men use the in-depth interview (or focus group) to reflect on personal histories that they attribute leading them to sexual risk taking, drug use, and an HIV or STI diagnosis (White et al., 2019). During these instances, it is crucial that interviewers show empathy and compassion and allow time for participants to share their perspective because an abrupt refocus on study goals could exacerbate research mistrust (DiCicco-Bloom & Crabtree, 2006). Interviewers must be prepared for emotional conversations during which participants may disclose histories of suicide ideation, childhood sexual abuse, resource instability, or drug and alcohol dependence, especially in sexual health prevention research with Black gay and bisexual men (Dickson-Swift et al., 2007). Additionally, protocols to refer and/or directly hand-offs participants to behavioral health services should be established and implemented when conducting in-depth interviews regarding sexual health among Black SMM. Allowing time and space for necessary probes along with providing the participant with an opportunity to share the information that is important to them. Although the in-depth interview is a research method and not a therapeutic session, Black SMM may be willing to share more information with researchers hey feel a genuine sense of care and understanding from the interviewer. This willingness to open up can lead to the collection of rich, nuanced data that is crucial for understanding the complexities of their experiences. However, it also places a significant responsibility on the interviewer to navigate these conversations with sensitivity, ensuring that the participant's emotional well-being is prioritized while maintaining the integrity and objectives of the research.

Focus Groups

Although in-depth qualitative interviews are useful to gather detailed, personal information regarding sensitive topics, focus groups utilize within-group perspectives, discussions, and interactions to elicit a range of perspectives from multiple participants simultaneously (Davidson et al., 2013; Happell, 2007). Focus groups are useful when the topics are general enough that people might be willing to share with others in a group. Focus groups have helped researchers uncover nuanced sociocultural experiences among Black SMM such as how racism, homonegativity, and stigma from society, family, and clinicians create barriers to HIV prevention behaviors (Cahill et al., 2017; Dangerfield II et al., 2018; White et al., 2019). In HIV/STI prevention science. Focus groups are also useful for designing and refining culturally relevant interventions (Dangerfield II et al., 2018, 2022a; Wilson et al., 2016). However, given the heterogeneity among Black SMM coupled with the fact that some of them have never shared their ideas or perspectives in a group or research setting, the protocols for focus group conduct for HIV/STI prevention research require more careful consideration, including the ways in which groups should be designed and conducted (White et al., 2019). Therefore, focus on sample size, facilitators, and facilitation in focus group methodology is needed.

Focus Group Sample Size

Focus group studies typically sample 8–12 participants per group for data collection until theoretical saturation is achieved (Hancock et al., 2016; Morse, 1995). However, smaller groups of between 5 and 7 might be more optimal for managing and eliciting rich data in prevention research with Black SMM (Dangerfield II et al., 2021b; White et al., 2019). Limiting the number of individuals in each group allows each participant to respond to every question in as much detail as possible without feeling rushed or fatigued by long meeting times. Obtaining detailed responses from everyone in the group allows researchers to gather a range of in-depth information and could enhance theoretical saturation. Moreover, it provides individuals who may have histories of being unheard or neglected with an opportunity to share their perspectives in a safe environment. In larger focus groups, there may be individuals who remain silent for most of the discussion and prevents researchers from obtaining optimal information from everyone in the group, especially in communities where mistrust is prevalent.

Limiting the number of individuals in the group can also increase participant comfort regarding privacy protection. The more people that are in the group, the greater opportunities there are for privacy breaches, regardless of informed consent and agreements among participants. Maintaining privacy is key to community engagement and building trust among Black SMM (Dangerfield II et al., 2021b; White et al., 2019). A smaller group is also more manageable for facilitators when disagreements arise between participants (Dangerfield II et al., 2021b; White et al., 2019). Although more focus groups may be required to obtain a large sample of study participants, researchers may find that theoretical saturation is achieved more efficiently within smaller groups because everyone in the group has the opportunity (and is encouraged) to respond to each question, which provides more data from everyone. Although the focus group leverages group dynamics to elicit data from participants, smaller groups can create a more intimate and supportive environment where participants feel safer to share personal and sensitive experiences, leading to richer and more authentic data among Black SMM. This environment fosters deeper discussions and more meaningful interactions, which are essential for understanding the complexities of sexual health and other sensitive topics among Black SMM. The increased sense of safety and intimacy can help mitigate the potential for power imbalances or dominance by more vocal participants (White et al., 2019), ensuring that all voices are heard and valued in the discussion.

Facilitating Focus Groups in Targeted HIV Research

Similar to in-depth interview conduct, focus groups should be facilitated by trained and trusted members of the community. Facilitators should also incorporate time for personal and group reflections during data collection and have sensibilities to transition in sensitive ways if the discussion gets off-topic from the primary research question(s). Of note, this is more feasible with a smaller group than a larger. Focus groups can be a space for particularly for participants (especially who are living with HIV) to share feelings about their marginalized and possibly traumatic experiences more than an opportunity to inform HIV interventions (White et al., 2019). Some older Black SMM who are living with HIV use the focus group to reflect on the past when they had limited social support, experienced social/religious stigma, and were vulnerable to sexual risk-taking behaviors (White et al., 2019). Some groups evolve into group therapy sessions rather than research data collection as members shared thoughts on how they could "heal themselves" rather than provide solutions to public health professionals (White et al., 2019). Since questions and comments about community-driven solutions increased during these kinds of reflections, I typically allow participants to share their feelings and were mindful to not abruptly transition the discussion back to the original goals of the research (White et al., 2019). This can lead to unique insights regarding community-drive solutions rather than researcher-driven solutions, which is aligned with qualitative methodology and contemporary intervention design frameworks (von Hippel, 2018; Wilson et al., 2016).

Still, culturally different interviewers should invest time in cultural competence training to understand the cultural context and sensitivities of the participants (Betancourt et al., 2003; Dangerfield II & Wylie, 2022). This helps interviewers to frame questions in culturally appropriate ways and recognize potential biases in their interpretations. Social support and interactions with others can help generate solutions for people with similar conditions, experiences, and circumstances. However, it is important to be mindful that the facilitator maintains a balance between allowing organic, therapeutic discussions and steering the conversation to meet the research objectives. This ensures that while participants' needs for emotional support are met, the primary goals of data collection are not compromised, ultimately enhancing the depth and relevance of the findings. Moreover, interviewers should continuously engage in self-reflection throughout the research process, evaluating how their own cultural background and personal experiences may influence their interactions with participants and the interpretation of the data (Jootun et al., 2009; Kanuha, 2000). This ongoing reflexivity, combined with active efforts to build rapport and trust with participants, can help mitigate potential cultural misunderstandings and foster a more open and productive dialogue, leading to richer, more nuanced insights that are genuinely reflective of the participants' perspectives (Dickson-Swift et al., 2007; Jootun et al., 2009).

Managing Health Status Discussions in Focus Group Settings

Prevention scientists should be mindful that for participants living with HIV, questions regarding HIV might not yield optimal data in the focus group context. For example, some Black SMM who are living with HIV might decline focus group participation immediately before group because they recognize others in the meeting and are uncomfortable discussing HIV-related issues in a group of familiar faces (White et al., 2019). Others could be reluctant to discuss issues regarding their HIV status despite knowing that they were meeting with other people living with HIV. Facilitators should continuously remind participants of the goals of the study, that the information they shared is confidential, and prepare participants for HIV-related questions if this method is chosen. Additionally, providing opportunities for private one-on-one interviews can be an effective alternative for those uncomfortable with group discussions. Ensuring a safe and supportive environment is crucial to obtaining honest and valuable insights from participants.

Managing Disagreements and Conflicts Within Groups

Disagreements can emerge when discussing sensitive information about attitudes toward community health, experiences, or negative interactions with healthcare organizations and community leaders. Especially because many people have not felt heard before. Therefore, managing disagreements or emotional upsets that may occur in the focus group context requires a nimble and iterative approach. Facilitators should be mindful of various levels of engagement, be able to manage group dynamics, and encourage full participation of group members. Specifically, facilitators should continuously remind participants that all opinions are welcomed and that information shared in the group should be respected and remain confidential. Managing disagreements is another reason why smaller focus groups are beneficial. To maintain rapport, decrease discomfort, and elicit optimal data, participants should consistently be reminded of the goals of the study and that information is confidential. While the presence of others enhances the richness of the data (Kitzinger, 1994, 2005), facilitators should be mindful of various levels of engagement, be able to manage group dynamics, and encourage full participation of group members. Facilitators should have the skills to manage disagreements during discussions and prepare participants for sensitive questions about HIV, sexuality, and possible histories of violence.

Online Synchronous Focus Groups

Virtual focus groups (i.e., focus groups that are not in-person) refer to online chatrooms, discussion boards, email correspondence (Adler & Zarchin, 2002; Murray, 1997), and more contemporary computer-mediated video communication modalities such as Zoom (Dodds & Hess, 2020; Rupert et al., 2017; Wirtz et al., 2019). Virtual, synchronous focus groups can provide a digital means to obtain qualitative data from several participants simultaneously (Adler & Zarchin, 2002; Sweet, 2001). Although conducting in-person focus groups is a popular approach for studies among Black SMM (Wilson et al., 2016), in-person research protocols are not always feasible. This was especially true when social distancing and stay-at-home orders were in place due to the COVID-19 quarantine in 2020. Conducting virtual focus groups can help researchers overcome various challenges related to study location, study costs, and obtaining perspectives from a range of community members (Stewart & Shamdasani, 2017; Woodyatt et al., 2016). Virtual focus groups can also reduce inhibitions and allow more free-flowing discussions because participants are likely in a more comfortable setting such as their home (Stewart &

Shamdasani, 2017). My work suggests that Black SMM men find virtual focus groups acceptable over in-person protocols and a preferred data collection method (Dangerfield II et al., 2021b). An intentional focus on privacy protocols, facilitation, and incentive distribution is needed for better engagement and data collection.

First, participants in virtual synchronous focus groups should be provided a password-protected Zoom link and instructed not to share the link with anyone. Once everyone joins the virtual focus group, the facilitator should ask each person to verbally confirm that they are in a private location to share and receive information. The facilitator should also confirm that they are in a private, IRB-approved location to build trust from the participants. Everyone (including facilitators) should confirm their privacy by showing participants their space on camera, unless individuals have headphones on (Dangerfield II et al., 2021b). Everyone should also confirm if they believe the study environment is safe enough to share their views virtually. Once the facilitator and participants determine the group's safety and privacy, the facilitator should lock the meeting using Zoom's "lock meeting" function and inform the participants that the meeting is locked. Participants should also be asked to change their Zoom screen name to an alternative (e.g., name of their favorite color) to limit the risk of a participant's given name being audio recorded or exposed in a computer screen shot. The research team should inform participants that if their location is compromised by another individual entering their space they would be removed from the virtual focus group and be prepared to do so (Dangerfield II et al., 2021b). Participants can also send private messages to the facilitator to express discomfort if needed. This level of detail useful to build trust among the participants and reinforces the commitment to confidentiality and safety, which is especially important when discussing sensitive topics like sexual health. Ensuring these protocols are followed helps to create a secure environment where participants feel comfortable sharing their experiences openly, ultimately leading to more authentic and valuable data collection.

Autoethnography

Autoethnography is a research method that uses the scientist's personal experiences to study and interpret cultural phenomena, offering a deeper understanding of cultural norms, values, emotions, and self-identity (Adams et al., 2017; Ellis et al., 2011). This approach provides insights that may be missed in other qualitative methods like interviews or focus groups, especially when participants view certain experiences as ordinary and do not discuss them. In HIV prevention research, autoethnography can reveal the complex challenges that hinder PrEP adoption among Black SMM, offering a nuanced understanding of personal identity and health issues in minority populations (Dangerfield II, 2023).

Conducting a high-quality autoethnography involves a combination of self-reflection, team members with whom you can be vulnerable, and rigorous analysis. Researchers should start by engaging in deep self-reflection, maintaining detailed journals to document personal experiences, thoughts, and emotions over time (Ellis et al., 2011; Tolich, 2010). This introspective process must be framed within existing academic literature and theories, enabling researchers to contextualize their personal narratives within broader cultural, social, or political frameworks. Transparency is essential; researchers need to clearly state their positionality and the lens through which they interpret their experiences, ensuring the reader understands their perspective (Chang, 2016; Kanuha, 2000; Tong et al., 2007). Balancing personal storytelling with critical analysis is crucial; personal anecdotes should be analyzed for their broader implications rather than merely recounted. Seeking feedback from peers and mentors can provide external perspectives that enhance the credibility and depth of the study (Chang, 2016). Ethical considerations are paramount; researchers must handle sensitive topics with care, ensuring confidentiality and respect for anyone mentioned in the narrative (Tolich, 2010). By integrating these elements, researchers can produce autoethnographies that are both deeply personal and academically robust.

I conducted autoethnography of my experiences as a PrEP using peer change agent in an intervention to improve perceived HIV risk among Black gay and bisexual men (Dangerfield II, 2023). This method's introspective nature enables researchers to contribute valuable personal insights that can enhance the design and implementation of public health interventions. By reflecting on my own experiences and challenges as a PrEP user and peer change agent, I was able to identify key factors that influence behavior change and adherence within the community. This approach also highlighted the importance of cultural competence and the need for tailored messaging that resonates with the experiences of Black gay and bisexual men. Ultimately, autoethnography provided a deeper understanding of the social dynamics and barriers to HIV prevention, offering practical recommendations for more effective and inclusive public health strategies.

Expanding on the use of autoethnography in my work, this approach also allowed for a deeper exploration of the intersections between personal identity, community engagement, and prevention messaging. By systematically studying and critically analyzing my experiences, I uncovered the nuanced ways in which stigma, community support, and personal empowerment intersect to shape health behaviors and decision-making among Black gay and bisexual men. This reflective process not only provided insights into individual experiences but also revealed broader systemic issues, such as the impact of healthcare access and the role of social networks in supporting or hindering HIV prevention efforts. Additionally, the autoethnographic approach facilitated the identification of gaps in existing interventions and the development of strategies that are more culturally responsive and effective. For instance, my reflections highlighted the importance of peer-led initiatives, where individuals with shared experiences can play a crucial role in educating and motivating others within the community. This method also underscored the need for ongoing dialogue and feedback loops between researchers and the communities they serve to ensure that interventions remain relevant and responsive to changing needs. I was able to offer a more holistic view of the challenges and opportunities in HIV prevention among Black gay and bisexual men with greater humanity, emphasizing the crucial role of community involvement and personal storytelling in shaping public health practices. The findings from this approach not only contribute to academic knowledge but also have practical implications for designing and implementing interventions that are grounded in the realities of those most affected by sexual health disparities.

Conclusions

Overall, qualitative research is feasible and acceptable and crucial for prevention science and intervention design for this group of racial and sexual minority men. Its ability to provide deep, contextual insights into human behavior and social dynamics, explore sensitive topics, inform tailored interventions, identify barriers and facilitators, contribute to theory development, and enhance quantitative research makes it a powerful tool in the pursuit of improved sexual health outcomes. However, careful consideration and attention to reflexivity and providing informed consent, ensuring privacy, data collection is necessary for optimal research. This chapter emphasizes the importance of culturally responsive qualitative methodologies in research involving Black SMM. It discusses various qualitative methods and how they can be adapted to respect and reflect the cultural contexts of participants, ensuring that research findings are both valid and relevant. Qualitative methodology plays a crucial role in prevention science for Black SMM by providing in-depth insights into their unique experiences, needs, and challenges. Through interviews, focus groups, and ethnographic studies, researchers can gather rich, detailed data that highlights the specific risk factors and protective factors relevant to these communities. This approach helps to uncover the underlying mechanisms of health disparities, informing the development of culturally sensitive and effective prevention interventions. By giving voice to those who might otherwise be overlooked or apprehensive, qualitative research ensures that the diversity of experiences is recognized and addressed in prevention efforts.

Raised Questions

1. How can prevention research ensure optimal data collection in qualitative research?
2. How can the qualitative researchers obtain high quality data among Black SMM?
3. What strategies can enhance the depth and richness of the data collected?

Chapter Summary

This chapter emphasized the crucial role of qualitative methodology in sexual health prevention science, particularly among Black SMM. Unlike quantitative methods, qualitative approaches provide rich, detailed data that capture the complexities of human behavior and social dynamics, making them essential for designing culturally responsive interventions. The chapter highlighted the importance of culturally competent and ethical qualitative research. It discussed various methods, such as in-depth interviews, focus groups, and autoethnography, and their application in understanding the specific needs and challenges faced by Black SMM. These methods allow researchers to gather personal and contextual data that might be overlooked in quantitative studies, offering deeper insights into the factors contributing to health disparities. The interviewer's role in qualitative research is key; culturally similar interviewers can establish trust and rapport more quickly, leading to more authentic and comprehensive data collection. Strategies for minimizing cultural barriers, such as cultural sensitivity training and ongoing reflexivity, were discussed as essential for enhancing data quality and ensuring that research findings are accurate and reflective of participants' true perspectives. Additionally, the chapter addresses the management of sensitive topics during interviews and focus groups, emphasizing the need for empathetic and skilled facilitators who can navigate difficult conversations while maintaining the research focus. The discussion on virtual focus groups and autoethnography demonstrates the adaptability of qualitative methods in various research contexts, including during the COVID-19 pandemic. In conclusion, this chapter suggested that qualitative research is indispensable for understanding and addressing the unique health challenges of Black SMM. It provides the necessary depth and context to inform the development of effective, culturally sensitive interventions.

Key Points

1. **The role and value of qualitative methodology in prevention science**: Qualitative research provides rich, in-depth insights into the behaviors, experiences, and contexts of marginalized communities such as Black SMM. Unlike quantitative methods, qualitative approaches allow researchers to explore complex social dynamics and personal narratives and contribute richly to effective, culturally responsive intervention designs.
2. **In-Depth Interviews**: In-depth interviews are a valuable method for collecting sensitive information in sexual health research. This method allows participants to share personal and potentially stigmatizing experiences, such as trauma or HIV status, in a private and safe environment. The role of the interviewer is crucial in managing sensitive discussions and maintaining trust throughout the interview process.
3. **Focus Groups**: Focus groups leverage group dynamics to elicit a range of perspectives. However, for research with Black SMM, smaller focus groups (5–7 participants) are recommended to ensure more intimate discussions, better privacy protection, and richer data. Facilitators should be skilled in managing group dynamics and sensitive topics to ensure that all participants are heard and that discussions remain focused on research goals.

4. **Virtual Focus Groups**: Virtual focus groups emerged as a practical alternative during the COVID-19 pandemic. They can reduce inhibitions and provide more flexibility for participants, making them a preferred method for some Black SMM. However, ensuring privacy and confidentiality in virtual settings is crucial, with detailed protocols to protect participants' identities and personal information.
5. **Autoethnography**: Autoethnography is a important qualitative method that uses the researcher's personal experiences to gain deeper insights into cultural phenomena. This method is particularly valuable in HIV prevention research, as it allows for a nuanced understanding of personal identity, community engagement, and health behaviors within marginalized communities such as Black SMM.
6. **Handling Sensitive Topics**: Both in-depth interviews and focus groups may involve discussing traumatic experiences, such as childhood abuse or HIV status. Researchers must be prepared to manage emotional conversations with empathy and compassion. Establishing protocols for referring participants to behavioral health services is also important to ensure their well-being during and after data collection.

References

Adams, T. E., Ellis, C., & Jones, S. H. (2017). Autoethnography. In *The International Encyclopedia of Communication Research Methods* (pp. 1–11). John Wiley & Sons, Ltd. https://doi.org/10.1002/9781118901731.iecrm0011

Adler, C. L., & Zarchin, Y. R. (2002). The "Virtual Focus Group": Using the internet to reach pregnant women on home bed rest. *Journal of Obstetric, Gynecologic, & Neonatal Nursing, 31*(4), 418–427. https://doi.org/10.1111/j.1552-6909.2002.tb00064.x

Arnold, E. A., Rebchook, G. M., & Kegeles, S. M. (2014). "Triply cursed": Racism, homophobia, and HIV-related stigma are barriers to regular HIV testing, treatment adherence, and disclosure among young Black gay men. *Culture, Health & Sexuality, 16*(6), 710–722. https://doi.org/10.1080/13691058.2014.905706

Betancourt, J. R., Green, A. R., Carrillo, J. E., & Ananeh-Firempong, O. (2003). Defining cultural competence: A practical framework for addressing racial/ethnic disparities in health and health care. *Public Health Reports®, 118*(4), 293–302. https://doi.org/10.1093/phr/118.4.293

Cahill, S., Taylor, S. W., Elsesser, S. A., Mena, L., Hickson, D., & Mayer, K. H. (2017). Stigma, medical mistrust, and perceived racism may affect PrEP awareness and uptake in black compared to white gay and bisexual men in Jackson, Mississippi and Boston, Massachusetts. *AIDS Care, 29*(11), 1351–1358. https://doi.org/10.1080/09540121.2017.1300633

Chang, H. (2016). *Autoethnography as method* (1st ed.). Routledge. https://doi.org/10.4324/9781315433370

Creswell, J. W., & Poth, C. N. (2016). *Qualitative inquiry and research design: Choosing among five approaches*. Sage.

Croot, E. J., Lees, J., & Grant, G. (2011). Evaluating standards in cross-language research: A critique of squires' criteria. *International Journal of Nursing Studies, 48*(8), 1002–1011. https://doi.org/10.1016/j.ijnurstu.2011.04.007

Dangerfield, D. T., II. (2023). A principal investigator as a PrEP-using peer change agent for HIV prevention among Black gay and bisexual men: An autoethnography. *International Journal*

of Environmental Research and Public Health, 20(7), Article 7. https://doi.org/10.3390/ijerph20075309
Dangerfield, D., II, & Wylie, C. (2022). Identifying ethical and culturally responsive research activities to build trust and improve participation of Black sexual minority men in pre-exposure prophylaxis telehealth clinical trials: Qualitative study. *JMIR Human Factors, 9*(1), e28798. https://doi.org/10.2196/28798
Dangerfield, D. T., II, Smith, L. R., Anderson, J. N., Bruce, O. J., Farley, J., & Bluthenthal, R. (2017). Sexual positioning practices and sexual risk among Black gay and bisexual men: A life course perspective. *AIDS and Behavior, 22*(6), 1919–1931. https://doi.org/10.1007/s10461-017-1948-6
Dangerfield, D. T., II, Harawa, N. T., McWells, C., Hilliard, C., & Bluthenthal, R. N. (2018). Exploring the preferences of a culturally congruent, peer-based HIV prevention intervention for black men who have sex with men. *Sexual Health, 15*(5), 424–430. https://doi.org/10.1071/SH18057
Dangerfield, D. T., II, Heidari, O., Cooper, J., Allen, S., & Lucas, G. M. (2020). Motivations for opioid and stimulant use among drug using black sexual minority men: A life course perspective. *Drug and Alcohol Dependence, 215*, 108224. https://doi.org/10.1016/j.drugalcdep.2020.108224
Dangerfield, D. T., II, Cooper, J., Heidari, O., Allen, S., Winder, T. J. A., & Lucas, G. M. (2021a). Nursing and health care preferences among opioid and stimulant using Black sexual minority men: An exploratory study. *Journal of the Association of Nurses in AIDS Care, 32*(5), e30–e39. https://doi.org/10.1097/JNC.0000000000000201
Dangerfield, D. T., II, Wylie, C., & Anderson, J. N. (2021b). Conducting virtual, synchronous focus groups among Black sexual minority men: Qualitative study. *JMIR Public Health and Surveillance, 7*(2), e22980. https://doi.org/10.2196/22980
Dangerfield, D. T., II, Anderson, J. N., Wylie, C., Arrington-Sanders, R., Bluthenthal, R. N., Beyrer, C., & Farley, J. E. (2022a). Refining a multicomponent intervention to increase perceived HIV risk and PrEP initiation: Focus group study among Black sexual minority men. *JMIR Formative Research, 6*(8), e34181. https://doi.org/10.2196/34181
Dangerfield, D. T., Lipson, A., & Anderson, J. N. (2022b). HIV PrEP clinician communication preferences among Black sexual minority men. *AIDS Education and Prevention, 34*(2), 168–181. https://doi.org/10.1521/aeap.2022.34.2.168
Davidson, P., Halcomb, E., & Gholizadeh, L. (2013). *Focus groups in health research.* Faculty of Science, Medicine and Health - Papers, 54–72.
della Porta, D. (2014). In-depth interviews. In *Methodological practices in social movement research.* Oxford University Press. https://edisciplinas.usp.br/pluginfile.php/8153942/course/section/6596823/DELLA%20PORTA.%20Methodological%20Practices%20in%20Social%20Movement%20Research-Oxford%20University%20Press%20%282014%29.pdf#page=243
DiCicco-Bloom, B., & Crabtree, B. F. (2006). The qualitative research interview. *Medical Education, 40*(4), 314–321. https://doi.org/10.1111/j.1365-2929.2006.02418.x
Dickson-Swift, V., James, E. L., Kippen, S., & Liamputtong, P. (2007). Doing sensitive research: What challenges do qualitative researchers face? *Qualitative Research, 7*(3), 327–353. https://doi.org/10.1177/1468794107078515
Dodds, S., & Hess, A. C. (2020). Adapting research methodology during COVID-19: Lessons for transformative service research. *Journal of Service Management, ahead-of-print* (ahead-of-print). https://doi.org/10.1108/JOSM-05-2020-0153
Dunbar, C., Rodriguez, D., & Laurence, L. (2002). Race, subjectivity, and the interview process. In *Handbook of interview research: Context and method.* Sage.
Ellis, C., Adams, T. E., & Bochner, A. P. (2011). Autoethnography: An overview. *Historical Social Research / Historische Sozialforschung, 36*(4 (138)), 273–290.
Gill, P., Stewart, K., Treasure, E., & Chadwick, B. (2008). Methods of data collection in qualitative research: Interviews and focus groups. *British Dental Journal, 204*(6), 291–295. https://doi.org/10.1038/bdj.2008.192

Guest, G., Namey, E., Taylor, J., Eley, N., & McKenna, K. (2017). Comparing focus groups and individual interviews: Findings from a randomized study. *International Journal of Social Research Methodology, 20*(6), 693–708. https://doi.org/10.1080/13645579.2017.1281601

Hancock, M. E., Amankwaa, L., Revell, M. A., & Coi, R. (2016). Focus group data saturation: A new approach to data analysis. *The Qualitative Report, 21*(11), 2124–2130.

Happell, B. (2007). Focus groups in nursing research: An appropriate method or the latest fad? *Nurse Researcher (through 2013); London, 14*(2), 18–24.

Jandt, F. E. (2017). *An introduction to intercultural communication: Identities in a global community*. Sage.

Johnson, J., & Rowlands, T. (2012). The interpersonal dynamics of in-depth interviewing. In *The SAGE handbook of interview research: The complexity of the craft*. Sage.

Johnstone, M.-L. (2017). Depth interviews and focus groups. In K. Kubacki & S. Rundle-Thiele (Eds.), *Formative research in social marketing: Innovative methods to gain consumer insights* (pp. 67–87). Springer. https://doi.org/10.1007/978-981-10-1829-9_5

Jootun, D., McGhee, G., & Marland, G. R. (2009). Reflexivity: Promoting rigour in qualitative research. *Nursing Standard (through 2013), 23*(23), 42–46.

Kanuha, V. K. (2000). "Being" native versus "going native": Conducting social work research as an insider. *Social Work, 45*(5), 439–447. https://doi.org/10.1093/sw/45.5.439

Kitzinger, J. (1994). The methodology of focus groups: The importance of interaction between research participants. *Sociology of Health & Illness, 16*(1), 103–121. https://doi.org/10.1111/1467-9566.ep11347023

Kitzinger, J. (2005). Focus group research: Using group dynamics to explore perceptions, experiences, and understandings. In *Qualitative research in health care* (pp. 56–68). McGraw-Hill Education (UK).

Liamputtong, P. (2010). *Performing qualitative cross-cultural research*. Cambridge University Press.

Morse, J. M. (1995). The significance of saturation. *Qualitative Health Research, 5*(2), 147–149. https://doi.org/10.1177/104973239500500201

Murray, P. J. (1997). Using virtual focus groups in qualitative research. *Qualitative Health Research, 7*(4), 542–549. https://doi.org/10.1177/104973239700700408

Quinn, K., Dickson-Gomez, J., Zarwell, M., Pearson, B., & Lewis, M. (2018). "A gay man and a doctor are just like, a recipe for destruction": How racism and homonegativity in healthcare settings influence PrEP uptake among young Black MSM. *AIDS and Behavior., 23*, 1951–1963. https://doi.org/10.1007/s10461-018-2375-z

Quinn, K., Bowleg, L., & Dickson-Gomez, J. (2019). "The fear of being Black plus the fear of being gay": The effects of intersectional stigma on PrEP use among young Black gay, bisexual, and other men who have sex with men. *Social Science & Medicine, 232*, 86–93. https://doi.org/10.1016/j.socscimed.2019.04.042

Rupert, D. J., Poehlman, J. A., Hayes, J. J., Ray, S. E., & Moultrie, R. R. (2017). Virtual versus in-person focus groups: Comparison of costs, recruitment, and participant logistics. *Journal of Medical Internet Research, 19*(3), e80. https://doi.org/10.2196/jmir.6980

Song, M., & Parker, D. (1995). Commonality, difference and the dynamics of disclosure in in-depth interviewing. *Sociology, 29*(2), 241–256. https://doi.org/10.1177/0038038595029002004

Stewart, D. W., & Shamdasani, P. (2017). Online focus groups. *Journal of Advertising, 46*(1), 48–60. https://doi.org/10.1080/00913367.2016.1252288

Sweet, C. (2001). Designing and conducting virtual focus groups. *Qualitative Market Research: An International Journal, 4*(3), 130–135. https://doi.org/10.1108/13522750110393035

Tolich, M. (2010). A critique of current practice: Ten foundational guidelines for autoethnographers. *Qualitative Health Research, 20*(12), 1599–1610. https://doi.org/10.1177/1049732310376076

Tong, A., Sainsbury, P., & Craig, J. (2007). Consolidated criteria for reporting qualitative research (COREQ): A 32-item checklist for interviews and focus groups. *International Journal for Quality in Health Care, 19*(6), 349–357. https://doi.org/10.1093/intqhc/mzm042

von Hippel, C. (2018). A next generation assets-based public health intervention development model: The public as innovators. *Frontiers in Public Health, 6*, 248. https://doi.org/10.3389/fpubh.2018.00248

White, J. J., Dangerfield, D. T., II, & Grieb, S. M. (2019). Methodological considerations for conducting focus groups in HIV prevention research among Black men who have sex with men. *Public Health Nursing, 36*(3), 439–445. https://doi.org/10.1111/phn.12592

Wilson, P. A., Valera, P., Martos, A. J., Wittlin, N. M., Muñoz-Laboy, M. A., & Parker, R. G. (2016). Contributions of qualitative research in informing HIV/AIDS interventions targeting Black MSM in the United States. *The Journal of Sex Research, 53*(6), 642–654. https://doi.org/10.1080/00224499.2015.1016139

Wirtz, A. L., Cooney, E. E., Chaudhry, A., Reisner, S. L., & Women (LITE), A. C. T. S. H. A. A. T. (2019). Computer-mediated communication to facilitate synchronous online focus group discussions: Feasibility study for qualitative HIV research among transgender women across the United States. *Journal of Medical Internet Research, 21*(3), e12569. https://doi.org/10.2196/12569

Woodyatt, C. R., Finneran, C. A., & Stephenson, R. (2016). In-person versus online focus group discussions: A comparative analysis of data quality. *Qualitative Health Research, 26*(6), 741–749. https://doi.org/10.1177/1049732316631510

Chapter 6
Peer Change Agents as Behavioral and Multilevel Interventionists

Chapter Objectives

1. Examine the role of peers in the lives and health outcomes of Black sexual minority men (SMM).
2. Identify how peer change agents (PCAs) can serve as behavioral and multilevel interventionists to support sexual health among Black SMM.
3. Identify best practices and challenges in utilizing PCAs as interventionists with Black SMM.

The Role of Peers Along the Life Course

A peer is someone who shares similar characteristics, experiences, or circumstances with another person. Some commonalities between peers include key characteristics such as age, ethnicity, cultural background, or life experiences; these and other in-group factors help establish a foundation of mutual understanding, relatability, and trust (McPherson et al., 2001). The essence of "peerness" lies in the equality and reciprocity of the relationship in which individuals can connect, communicate, and understand each other based on their similar experiences. Peers leverage their shared perspectives to establish trust, receive guidance, and obtain support (Mutchler & McDavitt, 2011; Pichon et al., 2022). Peer relationships are essential across the entire lifespan, contributing to various aspects of personal development (Antonucci et al., 2014; Steinberg & Morris, 2001) and are of crucial importance to the sexual health and quality of life of Black SMM (Arnold et al., 2018; Hermanstyne et al., 2018; White et al., 2020).

Peers play a significant role throughout the life course by influencing an individual's social, emotional, and cognitive development (Hartup, 1998), all of which

D. T. Dangerfield II, *Prevention Science & Targeted Methods for HIV/STI Research with Black Sexual Minority Men*,
https://doi.org/10.1007/978-3-031-85130-8_6

can affect disease prevention behaviors. From an early age, peers serve as a mirror through which people can see themselves and understand social behaviors, particularly from childhood into young adulthood. Adolescents rely heavily on peers to help form their identity and establish autonomy from parental figures (Steinberg & Morris, 2001), which is especially significant for Black SMM given the high prevalence of tenuous familial relationships and victimization in childhood (Dharma et al., 2024). Peers can shape health attitudes and prevention behaviors during adolescence and young adulthood (Kelly, 2004; Quinn et al., 2020; Steinberg & Morris, 2001). As individuals transition into adulthood, the role of peers evolves but remains significant. Adult peers play an important role in providing emotional/social support and guidance, which are vital for mental health, sexual health, and quality of life (Hermanstyne et al., 2018; O'Connor et al., 2011).

The Influence of Peers in the Lives of Black Sexual Minority Men

Peers play an essential role in the lives of Black SMM throughout their life course (Antonucci et al., 2014). First, they provide a crucial support system that fosters a sense of belonging and community, which is particularly important given the dual marginalization they experience due to both their racial and sexual identities. Peers also serve as a vital source of emotional support and resilience, offering a space where individuals can share experiences and strategies for coping with discrimination and stigma from family and society generally. For example, the House and Ball community, a subculture within the LGBTQ+ community that originated in the Harlem drag scene during the 1920s, is comprised of "houses" that function as surrogate families led by "mothers" and "fathers" who offer guidance, support, and mentorship to their "children" (Arnold & Bailey, 2009; Bailey, 2013). The houses compete in ballroom events, or "balls", that serve not only as a stage for artistic expression but also as safe spaces where members can navigate and celebrate their identities without experiencing discrimination from others outside of the community. This peer-based community provides crucial support by addressing issues such as homelessness, mental health, and sexual health (Arnold & Bailey, 2009). By offering a sense of belonging and validation, the House and Ball community empowers Black gay men to cope with the intersectional challenges of racism, homophobia, and marginalization, promoting their overall well-being and resilience (Arnold & Bailey, 2009; Kubicek et al., 2013). My research has similarly found that contemporary social networks within the house and ball community also support HIV treatment adherence using daily check-ins within iPhone group text messages (Dangerfield II et al., 2022b). This support is not limited to Black gay men who participate in the ballroom scene; it is just one example of how peers are supportive within the community and culture. Generally, these and other forms of support from peers helps Black gay and bisexual men navigate the challenges of intersectional stigma and discrimination and fosters self-efficacy, empowerment, and health behaviors (Quinn et al., 2020). Studies show that that peer-led interventions and support groups effectively promote safer sexual practices and reduce HIV incidence among Black SMM (Arnold et al., 2018; Simoni et al., 2011). Therefore, the role of peers extends beyond social support to include critical functions in health promotion and community resilience, underscoring their importance in the lives of Black SMM.

Given the fact that they are considered trusted sources of knowledge and guidance, peers also play a crucial role in health information sharing among Black SMM (Quinn et al., 2020). Due to stigma homophobia, and lack of culturally competent health information, Black SMM experience significant barriers to accessing relevant health information and quality healthcare, which contributes to medical mistrust, poor patient-clinician communication, and treatment non-adherence. For example, there is no formal platform or standardized curriculum (in schools or healthcare settings at least) for gay and bisexual adolescents and young adults to receive same-sex sexual health education with accurate information besides general information regarding condom use. Therefore, Black SMM find a safe space to express their identities, share personal narratives, and seek advice without fear of judgment within peer networks (Quinn et al., 2020). Peers provide a culturally sensitive and relatable platform for sharing information, including sexual health education, HIV prevention strategies, and mental health resources (Barrington et al., 2009; Dangerfield II et al., 2022a; Quinn et al., 2020). By fostering open discussions, sharing personal stories, and offering practical advice, peers can translate health information relative to social and cultural experiences and influence health behaviors (Arnold et al., 2018; Dangerfield II & Anderson, 2024; Kelly, 2004; Quinn et al., 2020). Given the lack of formal sexual health education for sexual minority populations, this information is not always correct. An intentional focus on sexual health misinformation will be discussed in Chap. 9. However, peers are trusted sources of information, guidance because of they have shared experiences, and mutual trust, making health messages more relevant, credible, and effective. The support provided by peers includes emotional encouragement, resource sharing, and health information dissemination, bridging the gap created by shortcomings in mainstream society and healthcare to address the unique challenges faced by Black SMM.

Peer Change Agents

Peer change agents (PCAs) are lay individuals who can utilize their shared social identities and experiences to influence health behaviors within their communities (Dangerfield II, 2023; Schneider et al., 2015; Young et al., 2017). PCAs are trained to disseminate health information in communities in which they are members to facilitate behavior change (Dangerfield II & Anderson, 2024; Weeks et al., 2009; Young et al., 2017). PCAs are particularly effective in engaging communities in which social marginalization and medical mistrust are prevalent because they may have experienced and overcome similar social challenges and barriers to the behaviors they are promoting (Dangerfield II et al., 2018, 2022a; Quinn et al., 2020). PCA disclosure of personal and clinical experiences such as PrEP use, experiences of marginalization, or relationship challenges could be an important component that contributed to the effectiveness of peer-based approaches generally (Dangerfield II et al., 2018, 2022a). Black SMM may value personal disclosures because they believe researchers and clinicians lack understanding of their experiences and have insufficient knowledge of side effects and efficacy (Cahill et al., 2017; Dangerfield II et al., 2021, 2022a; Quinn et al., 2018). Additionally, they feel clinicians often fail to communicate in a way that is easily understood. Interventions using PCAs have changed community health beliefs and increased the uptake of HIV testing, PrEP, and adherence to antiretroviral therapy among different vulnerable populations, including Black SMM (Dangerfield II & Anderson, 2024; Weeks et al., 2009; Young et al., 2017). These interventions leverage the credibility and relatability of peers to deliver tailored health messages, foster open discussions about safe sex practices, and provide emotional support. The success of PCA-based interventions underscores the critical role that peer support plays in addressing health disparities and promoting behavior change within marginalized communities.

Focus on PCAs in HIV/STI prevention science is important for several reasons. First, heir relatable experiences make them more effective in communicating health messages and influencing behavior change, especially among minority communities. Additionally, using PCAs in interventions can improve recruitment and community engagement in research and health behaviors (see Chap. 3). Moreover, PCAs possess a deep understanding of the cultural norms, values, and beliefs of the community they serve and can bridge knowledge and communication gaps between researchers, clinicians, and Black SMM (Dangerfield II, 2023; Dangerfield II et al., 2022a; Dangerfield II & Anderson, 2024). PCAs can also reveal implementation scientific challenges that could impact research participation, uptake of prevention behaviors, and intervention effects. PCAs in HIV/STI prevention science is vital for effectively addressing the unique needs of minority communities. Their involvement not only enhances communication and trust but also strengthens the overall impact and sustainability of interventions, ultimately contributing to better health outcomes and more inclusive research practices.

Key Differences Between Peer Change Agents and Community Health Workers

Healthcare and social service models are increasing leveraging the role of cultural similarities and community connection into health professionalism and staffing structures using community health workers (CHW). CHWs are trusted community members who act as a bridge between healthcare services and the community and provide health education, support, and patient advocacy to improve healthcare access and enhance the quality of service delivery (Olaniran et al., 2017). CHWs conduct outreach, offer informal counseling, and patient navigation (Farley et al., 2021; Olaniran et al., 2017). Similar to PCAs, CHWs are often members of the communities they serve, which enhances their ability to build trust, understand cultural nuances, and effectively communicate health information (Pérez & Martinez, 2008). Studies have shown that CHWs can lead to significant improvements in health behaviors and outcomes, particularly in chronic disease management and preventive care across cultural contexts (Berini et al., 2022; Kim et al., 2016; Viswanathan et al., 2010). CHW models first gained traction in Latin America during the 1960s and 1970s, notably with Brazil's community health agent program and Mexico's "promotoras" initiatives, which employed local individuals who understood the cultural and social contexts of their communities to address health issues in rural and marginalized areas (Lehmann & Sanders, 2007). In the United States, the CHW model emerged during the War on Poverty in the 1960s, with programs such as the Neighborhood Health Center and migrant health initiatives incorporating CHWs to bridge gaps between healthcare systems and the populations they served (Brownstein et al., 2011; Olaniran et al., 2019). Over time, the CHW model has evolved and expanded globally, integrating into formal healthcare systems while retaining its foundational principles of community engagement, cultural competence, and grassroots advocacy (Olaniran et al., 2017, 2019). Today, CHWs are recognized by the World Health Organization as essential contributors to public health, particularly in addressing social determinants of health and improving healthcare access for vulnerable populations (World Health Organization, 2018).

PCAs and CHWs are both trained professionals who share similar demographic and cultural characteristics with community members and disseminate accurate health information to improve health care engagement (Farley et al., 2021; Schneider et al., 2015; Young et al., 2017).. However, they differ in several key aspects related to their identities, roles, training, and scope of work. Specifically, PCAs are typically members of the specific community they serve, sharing similar experiences, backgrounds, and identities with their "clients" (or peers). Their shared identity fosters trust and perceived support quickly and influences behavior because they may be recruited directly from the community to support health interventions within their social networks. Their primary role is to leverage their experiences to educate, support, and advocate for their peers, often in informal (i.e., community based or digital) settings. In contrast, contemporary CHW (especially in the U.S.) are generally trained professionals who may not necessarily share the all of the same characteristics or experiences as the individuals they serve. Additionally, CHWs undergo formal training and certification processes to gain a broad understanding of health issues, healthcare systems, and intervention strategies (O'Brien et al., 2009). They often work in more structured environments than PCAs, who often work as research interventionists, and may be involved in a wider range of activities, including clinical tasks, health education, case management, and connecting individuals to healthcare services. While both roles are crucial, PCAs excel in community-specific outreach and personalized support, whereas CHWs provide a broader, more formalized range of health services and support within healthcare environments. However, the PCA role is currently not a formal job within healthcare settings and cannot be executed properly by individuals without training in intervention design, motivational interviewing techniques, or research ethics. PCAs must also be comfortable with disclosing personal information, which could be key to building trust in PrEP among hesitant minority community members but raises some ethical questions regarding healthcare professionalism (Brownstein et al., 2011; Dangerfield II, 2023).

PCAs may be particularly effective at improving HIV prevention behavior among Black SMM because their prior experiences navigating PrEP barriers enhance their perceived trustworthiness (Dangerfield II et al., 2022a; Young et al., 2017). However, CHW protocols are often nebulous or missing and few focus on racial and sexual minority communities (Dangerfield II et al., 2023; Farley et al., 2021). Therefore, it is difficult to understand what health information is communicated within the community, how CHWs (or PCAs) address barriers, or how to replicate their health communication protocol across community contexts. The lack of clear CHW protocols tailored to Black SMM communities poses a challenge. Addressing these gaps is essential for standardizing health communication, effectively overcoming multilevel barriers, and ensuring the replicability of successful interventions across different community contexts.

PCAs as Behavioral Interventionists

The Introduction to this handbook described how behavioral interventions for sexual health prevention research aim to change risk taking behaviors using a variety of methods including education and awareness, skill-building, and motivational techniques. PCAs can function as effective behavioral interventionists by leveraging their shared experiences and cultural understanding to do each of these things in culturally responsive and acceptable ways. As individuals who often come from the same demographic and social backgrounds as the target population, they are uniquely positioned to understand the specific barriers and motivators that affect behavior change. Collectively, the literature on peers as behavioral interventionists in HIV prevention among Black SMM underscores the efficacy and importance of peer-led interventions in reducing HIV transmission rates and promoting sexual health within this community. Some HIV prevention studies have utilized PCAs to communicate health information, provide emotional support, and promote health behaviors (Dangerfield II & Anderson, 2024; Weeks et al., 2009; Young et al., 2017). PCAs have improved sexual health behaviors uptake partly because they can quickly create a supportive environment that fosters trust and open communication, making it easier for individuals to discuss their health concerns and challenges.

PCAs can also enhance knowledge and changes attitudes towards HIV prevention such as HIV testing and PrEP but also empowers individuals to accept recommendations to adopt healthier behaviors, thus demonstrating a significant positive impact on the overall health outcomes of Black SMM. They are also sometimes considered more trustworthy than clinicians when they can educate peers about health risks and prevention strategies, model health behaviors, and facilitate access to resources and services (Dangerfield II et al., 2018, 2021, 2022a). Through these efforts, PCAs not only promote immediate behavior change but cam also contribute to long-term health improvements and the overall well-being of their communities.

Peer Change Agents as Multilevel Interventionists

Remember from the Introduction of this handbook that multilevel interventions in HIV/STI prevention research focus on changing the multiple socioecological factors, including individual behavioral factors as well as broader social and/or environmental factors that influence disease risk, prevention and treatment services, and health outcomes (Brown et al., 2019; Phillips et al., 2021). PCAs can be considered multilevel interventionists in HIV/STI prevention for several novel reasons. First, they play a crucial role in enhancing social support networks and advocating for the needs of their peers, thereby creating a more supportive environment that facilitates health behaviors and access to prevention and treatment resources. Additionally, their in-group membership, shared experiences of marginalization, and trusted communication can also address systemic barriers such as stigma, discrimination, and mistrust of healthcare systems that prevent Black SMM from accessing services. Importantly, PCAs can alter the typical structures of clinical environments and healthcare policy by adding support staff within healthcare systems to serve several important functions including sharing trustworthy health information and destigmatizing prevention behaviors (including PrEP use). Potentially, PCAs could serve as a liaison between marginalized community members and clinicians (Dangerfield II et al., 2022a), which has been done in oncology research and practice (Eggly et al., 2006; Street & Gordon, 2008) but remains underutilized in the sexual health prevention landscape. My research suggests that having another Black SMM to discuss sexual health before visiting a clinician is acceptable if he was relatable and trustworthy (Dangerfield II et al., 2022a). As a supportive staff member in healthcare environments, a PCA could both dismantle misinformation and stigma for peers and help convey the needs of patients to clinicians, which could be crucial for circumventing medical mistrust and discriminatory clinical practices. Data show that clinicians are more likely to have prejudice, stigma, and discriminatory prescription practices towards Black SMM than white SMM (Adams & Balderson, 2016; Beer et al., 2016; Calabrese et al., 2018; Quinn et al., 2018). Therefore, PCAs can advocate on behalf of the needs of patients to circumvent the impacts of these structural factors within the healthcare setting, ensuring that services are more responsive and respectful. PCAs can help to dismantle structural impediments to health by working to change the social dynamics within their communities and institutional practices within healthcare settings, making them a vital, novel, and effective component of multilevel public health interventions. However, some Black SMM also mention concerns that working with a PCA prior to visiting a clinician could be another barrier that does not necessarily address racism and stigma (Dangerfield II et al., 2022a).

POSSIBLE: A Multicomponent intervention to Improve Perceived HIV Risk and PrEP Willingness among Black Gay and Bisexual Men

PCAs may be particularly effective at improving HIV prevention behavior among Black SMM because their prior experiences navigating PrEP barriers enhance their perceived trustworthiness (Dangerfield II et al., 2022a; Young et al., 2017). However, CHW protocols are often nebulous or missing and few focus on racial and sexual minority communities (Dangerfield II et al., 2023; Farley et al., 2021). Therefore, it is difficult to understand what health information is communicated within the community, how PCAs and CHWs address multilevel barriers, or how to replicate their health communication protocol across community contexts (Dangerfield II et al., 2023; Farley et al., 2021).

POSSIBLE was a theoretically guided intervention that incorporated a PCA who was matched with participants' key demographic and cultural characteristics based upon formative research identifying preferences among Black SMM (Dangerfield II et al., 2018, 2022a). The premise behind the intervention was to improve perceived HIV risk as a key cognitive precursor to PrEP initiation. Briefly, the intervention involved two virtual sessions with a PrEP-using PCA who used a script to assess participants' goals, values, and risks, share prevention information, and encourage PrEP use. Given my formative research and explicit recommendations from the community, I used PrEP and served the intervention as the PCA for 2 years (Dangerfield II, 2023). Participants also downloaded a publicly available app called PrEPme to record their sexual risk behaviors in an app-based diary for a month then reviewed the diary with the PCA (myself) to reassess their PrEP interest in the second session. Baseline results also showed a statistically significant difference in PRH after the first session with the PCA (Dangerfield II & Anderson, 2024). After baseline sessions, almost participants were willing to be referred to PrEP services; 69% of those confirmed scheduled appointments with PrEP care teams.

This suggests that the scripted PCA can help individuals whose behaviors confer greater risk for HIV understand their relative risks and catalyze behavior change. The PCA gently guides participants to identify discrepancies between their behaviors and HIV goals without stigma and activates intrinsic motivations, demonstrated by satisfaction scores. Providing adequate health information and tailoring prevention messaging to help Black SMM understand the relative risk of their behaviors could be key to this shift. Moreover, the peerness aspect of the intervention—the shared experiences and identity between the PCA and participants—was integral to its success. It allowed for a deeper connection, fostering an environment where participants felt understood and supported by someone who shared similar challenges and goals. This element of peerness not only enhanced the relevance and impact of the intervention but also contributed to building a sustainable model for future sexual health prevention strategies within marginalized communities.

The PCA model in POSSIBLE is highly significant because rather than generically relying upon sociodemographic characteristics (being Black, gay, or a resident in the community) to engage community and help patients navigate the healthcare system, POSSIBLE created a foundation for using a PCA to address sexual health barriers in a more systematic way. With the PCA model, researchers can better identify the points of intervention effects and replicate this approach because of the scripted nature of the interactions, even though they are tailored at the end. Interventions using community health worker or motivational interviewing approaches often have nebulous or (missing) protocols that make it difficult to replicate or scale across multiple contexts (Dangerfield II et al., 2023). It also better guided more sociological understandings of peerness and minority health promotion by (1) systematically identifying preferences for PCA characteristics from Black gay men and (2) leveraging ideal characteristics and health communication to improve perceived risks in a culturally responsive way.

Identifying Key Aspects of Peerness Necessary for Effective Interventions

Overall, my research suggests that key aspects of peerness among Black SMM revolve around the concepts of shared identity, vulnerable or marginalized experiences, and cultural familiarity to quickly build trust (Dangerfield II et al., 2022a; Dangerfield II & Wylie, 2022). For examples, studies indicate that interventionists who engage Black SMM should be Black, identify with the LGBT+ community, and have similar experiences such as navigating interactions with romantic or sexual partners, clinicians, and socio-economic challenges (Dangerfield II et al., 2018, 2021, 2022a). Additionally, the interventionist (or PCA) should also have overcome social and psychological challenges and be a "future self" to whom Black SMM could aspire (Dangerfield II et al., 2018, 2022a). Moreover, data show that PCAs promoting biomedical HIV prevention strategies should be a current PrEP user so they could share their experiences with side effects and maintaining adherence (Dangerfield II et al., 2022a). Black SMM suggest that similarities in life experiences are important to prevention scientists understanding of the challenging and complex circumstances of racial and sexual minority clients. These elements of peerness are characterized by a deep sense of solidarity, compassion, and support formed through common experiences of racial and sexual marginalization. These and other characteristics such as aesthetics (e.g., style of dress), language use, personal disclosures, and neighborhood familiarity serve as indicators for Black SMM to use to anticipate how stigmatizing, trustworthy, or relatable the PCA would be (Dangerfield II et al., 2022a).

Studies also indicate age-related differences in preferences for peer characteristics regarding additional PCA characteristics and the practical role of the PCA (Dangerfield II et al., 2018, 2022a). For example, young Black SMM share preferences for having a PCA was older or a Black woman, partly due to anticipated within-group stigma from in-group members who might judge their sexual behaviors as risky (Dangerfield II et al., 2022a). This is significant because under the classic understandings of peer-based models, these preferences (older, woman, heterosexual) may not easily fit into definitions of peerness and require further study. Data also indicate that that some older Black SMM prefer not to engage with a PCA in practice because they did not want to relieve clinicians of the responsibility of asking detailed and personal questions to know them as patients (Dangerfield II et al., 2022a), even though they believe a PCA should be a Black SMM. More research is needed to better understand the nuances of peer preferences and to refine the role and characteristics of PCAs to meet the diverse needs of Black SMM effectively. The relevant impact of these preferences should also be formally tested in interventions.

Conclusions

Peers play a crucial role in the lives and health outcomes among Black SMM and could be effectively leveraged as change agents for sexual health promotion if adequately utilized and scaled. As members of the community, PCAs possess a deep understanding of the cultural and social contexts that shape attitudes and behaviors regarding sexual health. They can effectively address stigma and misinformation related to HIV and PrEP, which are common barriers in this population. Their shared experiences and trust within the community make them credible sources of information, thereby enhancing the likelihood of successful health interventions. By fostering open communication and providing tailored education, PCAs can promote safer sex practices, encourage regular HIV testing, and facilitate the adoption of preventive measures like PrEP. This peer-led approach not only empowers individuals but also strengthens community resilience and engagement in sexual health initiatives, leading to more sustainable health outcomes.

Raised Questions

1. What are the key aspects that define effective peer-based strategies in HIV/STI prevention science interventions for Black SMM?
2. Who qualifies to be the peer change agent in interventions, and what criteria or processes should be used to select interventionists?
3. Which specific characteristics of "peerness" are most effective for conveying accurate health information to Black SMM?

Chapter Summary

This chapter explored the crucial role that peers play in the health outcomes of Black SMM. The chapter highlighted how peers, defined by shared experiences and characteristics, contribute significantly to the development and health behaviors of individuals across the life course. The chapter emphasized the importance of peer relationships in providing emotional support, fostering a sense of community, and influencing health behaviors. A central theme is the role of peer change agents (PCAs) in HIV/STI prevention, particularly among Black SMM. PCAs, who share similar social identities and experiences with the communities they serve, were discussed as effective behavioral and multilevel interventionists. For example, they are uniquely positioned to build trust and credibility, making them particularly effective in promoting health behaviors like HIV testing and PrEP adherence. The chapter also discusses the differences between PCAs and community health workers (CHWs), noting that although both play essential roles in health promotion, PCAs leverage personal experiences and cultural knowledge to address specific community needs. This chapter underscores the effectiveness of peer-led interventions and the need for further research to refine the role of PCAs, particularly regarding age-related preferences and the nuances of "peerness". In conclusion, the chapter raises questions about the key characteristics that make peer strategies effective, the criteria for selecting PCAs, and the specific aspects of "peerness" that are most impactful in conveying health information to Black SMM. The insights provided suggest that PCAs are vital in fostering community engagement in sexual health initiatives and could be key to supporting more sustainable health outcomes in the community.

Key Points

1. **The role of peers along the life course**: Peers, defined by shared characteristics and experiences, play a crucial role throughout the life course of Black SMM. Peer relationships provide emotional and social support, help shape identity, and influence health behaviors. These connections are essential for Black SMM as they navigate intersectional challenges regarding racism, homophobia, and marginalization.
2. **Peer change agents (PCAs)**: PCAs are individuals who use their shared social identities and experiences to influence health behaviors within their communities. As trusted in-group sources, they disseminate health information, promote behavior change, and help overcome barriers like medical mistrust in the community. PCAs have been effective in improving HIV prevention behaviors, such as increasing HIV testing, PrEP initiation, and HIV treatment adherence among Black SMM. PCAs can build trust and credibility in medicine and health care recommendations, which is crucial for addressing social barriers.

3. **Key differences between peer change agents (PCAs) and community health workers)**: Although both PCAs and CHWs are trusted community members who provide health education and support, PCAs are more focused on leveraging shared identities and experiences to connect with their peers. CHWs, on the other hand, typically undergo formal training and may not share the same level of personal experience with the community they serve. PCAs are often more effective in informal, community-based settings. More research is needed to identify the requisite social characteristics required for effective engagement for both PCAs and CHWs.
4. **PCAs as behavioral and multilevel interventionists**: PCAs can function as both behavioral interventionists, by promoting individual behavior change, and multilevel interventionists, by also addressing social and structural factors within healthcare settings. They help improve health behaviors, challenge misinformation, and reduce stigma. Additionally, PCAs can facilitate policy changes within healthcare systems to make services more responsive to the needs of Black SMM.
5. **Challenges and best practices with peer-based studies**: Successful PCA interventions require careful consideration of the characteristics that define "peerness" and how these characteristics influence health communication. Key aspects of effective PCAs include shared identity, experiences of marginalization, and cultural familiarity. Research suggests that these elements help PCAs build trust quickly, making them more effective in promoting health behaviors.
6. **Future research and refinement**: There is a need for further research to refine the role of PCAs, particularly in understanding age-related preferences and the nuances of "peerness." As interventions are developed, it is essential to identify which specific characteristics make PCAs most effective in conveying health information and driving behavior change among Black SMM.

References

Adams, L. M., & Balderson, B. H. (2016). HIV providers' likelihood to prescribe pre-exposure prophylaxis (PrEP) for HIV prevention differs by patient type: A short report. *AIDS Care, 28*(9), 1154–1158. https://doi.org/10.1080/09540121.2016.1153595

Antonucci, T. C., Ajrouch, K. J., & Birditt, K. S. (2014). The convoy model: Explaining social relations from a multidisciplinary perspective. *The Gerontologist, 54*(1), 82–92. https://doi.org/10.1093/geront/gnt118

Arnold, E. A., & Bailey, M. M. (2009). Constructing home and family: How the ballroom community supports African American GLBTQ youth in the face of HIV/AIDS. *Journal of Gay & Lesbian Social Services, 21*(2–3), 171–188. https://doi.org/10.1080/10538720902772006

Arnold, E. A., Sterrett-Hong, E., Jonas, A., & Pollack, L. M. (2018). Social networks and social support among ball-attending African American men who have sex with men and transgender women are associated with HIV-related outcomes. *Global Public Health, 13*(2), 144–158. https://doi.org/10.1080/17441692.2016.1180702

Bailey, M. M. (2013). *Butch Queens up in pumps: Gender, performance, and ballroom culture in Detroit*. University of Michigan Press.

Barrington, C., Latkin, C., Sweat, M. D., Moreno, L., Ellen, J., & Kerrigan, D. (2009). Talking the talk, walking the walk: Social network norms, communication patterns, and condom use among the male partners of female sex workers in La Romana, Dominican Republic. *Social Science & Medicine, 68*(11), 2037–2044. https://doi.org/10.1016/j.socscimed.2009.03.009

Beer, L., Bradley, H., Mattson, C. L., Johnson, C. H., Hoots, B., & Shouse, R. L. (2016). Trends in racial and ethnic disparities in antiretroviral therapy prescription and viral suppression in the United States, 2009–2013. *Journal of Acquired Immune Deficiency Syndromes (1999), 73*(4), 446–453. https://doi.org/10.1097/QAI.0000000000001125

Berini, C. R., Bonilha, H. S., & Simpson, A. N. (2022). Impact of community health workers on access to care for rural populations in the United States: A systematic review. *Journal of Community Health, 47*(3), 539–553. https://doi.org/10.1007/s10900-021-01052-6

Brown, A. F., Ma, G. X., Miranda, J., Eng, E., Castille, D., Brockie, T., Jones, P., Airhihenbuwa, C. O., Farhat, T., Zhu, L., & Trinh-Shevrin, C. (2019). Structural interventions to reduce and eliminate health disparities. *American Journal of Public Health, 109*(S1), S72–S78. https://doi.org/10.2105/AJPH.2018.304844

Brownstein, J. N., Hirsch, G. R., Rosenthal, E. L., & Rush, C. H. (2011). Community health workers "101" for primary care providers and other stakeholders in health care systems. *The Journal of Ambulatory Care Management, 34*(3), 210–220. https://doi.org/10.1097/JAC.0b013e31821c645d

Cahill, S., Taylor, S. W., Elsesser, S. A., Mena, L., Hickson, D., & Mayer, K. H. (2017). Stigma, medical mistrust, and perceived racism may affect PrEP awareness and uptake in black compared to white gay and bisexual men in Jackson, Mississippi and Boston, Massachusetts. *AIDS Care, 29*(11), 1351–1358. https://doi.org/10.1080/09540121.2017.1300633

Calabrese, S. K., Earnshaw, V. A., Krakower, D. S., Underhill, K., Vincent, W., Magnus, M., Hansen, N. B., Kershaw, T. S., Mayer, K. H., Betancourt, J. R., & Dovidio, J. F. (2018). A closer look at racism and hterosexism in medical students' clinical decision-making related to HIV pre-exposure prophylaxis (PrEP): Implications for PrEP education. *AIDS and Behavior, 22*(4), 1122–1138. https://doi.org/10.1007/s10461-017-1979-z

Dangerfield, D. T., II. (2023). A principal investigator as a PrEP-using peer change agent for HIV prevention among Black gay and bisexual men: An autoethnography. *International Journal of Environmental Research and Public Health, 20*(7), Article 7. https://doi.org/10.3390/ijerph20075309

Dangerfield, D. T., II, & Anderson, J. N. (2024). A scripted, PrEP-using peer change agent improves perceived risk for HIV and willingness to accept referrals quickly among Black sexual minority men: Preliminary findings from POSSIBLE. *AIDS and Behavior., 28*, 2156–2165. https://doi.org/10.1007/s10461-024-04313-2

Dangerfield, D., II, & Wylie, C. (2022). Identifying ethical and culturally responsive research activities to build trust and improve participation of Black sexual minority men in pre-exposure prophylaxis telehealth clinical trials: Qualitative study. *JMIR Human Factors, 9*(1), e28798. https://doi.org/10.2196/28798

Dangerfield, D. T., II, Harawa, N. T., McWells, C., Hilliard, C., & Bluthenthal, R. N. (2018). Exploring the preferences of a culturally congruent, peer-based HIV prevention intervention for black men who have sex with men. *Sexual Health, 15*(5), 424–430. https://doi.org/10.1071/SH18057

Dangerfield, D. T., II, Cooper, J., Heidari, O., Allen, S., Winder, T. J. A., & Lucas, G. M. (2021). Nursing and health care preferences among opioid and stimulant using Black sexual minority men: An exploratory study. *Journal of the Association of Nurses in AIDS Care, 32*(5), e30–e39. https://doi.org/10.1097/JNC.0000000000000201

Dangerfield, D. T., II, Anderson, J. N., Wylie, C., Arrington-Sanders, R., Bluthenthal, R. N., Beyrer, C., & Farley, J. E. (2022a). Refining a multicomponent intervention to increase perceived HIV risk and PrEP initiation: Focus group study among Black sexual minority men. *JMIR Formative Research, 6*(8), e34181. https://doi.org/10.2196/34181

Dangerfield, D. T., II, Ober, A. J., Li, M. J., Allen, S., & Bluthenthal, R. N. (2022b). HIV treatment adherence strategies among virally suppressed Black sexual minority men in Baltimore, Maryland, and Los Angeles, California: A theory-based qualitative study. *Journal of the Association of Nurses in AIDS Care, 33*(1), 54–62. https://doi.org/10.1097/JNC.0000000000000304

Dangerfield, D. T., II, Davis, G., Pandian, V., & Anderson, J. N. (2023). Using motivational interviewing to increase HIV PrEP initiation and adherence: A scoping review. *Prevention Science., 24*, 1365–1375. https://doi.org/10.1007/s11121-023-01554-w

Dharma, C., Keyes, K. M., Rudolph, K. E., Shrader, C.-H., Chen, Y.-T., Schneider, J., & Duncan, D. T. (2024). Adverse childhood experiences among Black sexually minoritized men and Black transgender women in Chicago. *International Journal for Equity in Health, 23*(1), 74. https://doi.org/10.1186/s12939-024-02168-6

Eggly, S., Penner, L. A., Greene, M., Harper, F. W. K., Ruckdeschel, J. C., & Albrecht, T. L. (2006). Information seeking during "bad news" oncology interactions: Question asking by patients and their companions. *Social Science & Medicine, 63*(11), 2974–2985. https://doi.org/10.1016/j.socscimed.2006.07.012

Farley, J. E., Dangerfield, D. T., II, LaRicci, J., Sacamano, P., Heidari, O., Lowensen, K., Jennings, J. M., & Tobin, K. E. (2021). Community engagement and linkage to care efforts by peer community-health workers to increase PrEP uptake among sexual minority men. *Public Health Nursing, 38*(5), 818–824. https://doi.org/10.1111/phn.12887

Hartup, W. (1998). The company they keep: Friendships and their developmental significance. In *The social child* (1st ed., pp. 143–163). Psychology Press. https://doi.org/10.4324/9781315784748-8

Hermanstyne, K. A., Green, H. D., Cook, R., Tieu, H.-V., Dyer, T. V., Hucks-Ortiz, C., Wilton, L., Latkin, C., & Shoptaw, S. (2018). Social network support and decreased risk of seroconversion in Black MSM: Results of the BROTHERS (HPTN 061) study. *Journal of Acquired Immune Deficiency Syndromes (1999), 78*(2), 163–168. https://doi.org/10.1097/QAI.0000000000001645

Kelly, J. A. (2004). Popular opinion leaders and HIV prevention peer education: Resolving discrepant findings, and implications for the development of effective community programmes. *AIDS Care, 16*(2), 139–150. https://doi.org/10.1080/09540120410001640986

Kim, K., Choi, J. S., Choi, E., Nieman, C. L., Joo, J. H., Lin, F. R., Gitlin, L. N., & Han, H.-R. (2016). Effects of community-based health worker interventions to improve chronic disease management and care among vulnerable populations: A systematic review. *American Journal of Public Health, 106*(4), e3–e28. https://doi.org/10.2105/AJPH.2015.302987

Kubicek, K., McNeeley, M., Holloway, I. W., Weiss, G., & Kipke, M. D. (2013). "It's like our own little world": Resilience as a factor in participating in the ballroom community subculture. *AIDS and Behavior, 17*(4), 1524–1539. https://doi.org/10.1007/s10461-012-0205-2

Lehman, U., & Sanders, D. (2007). Community health workers: what do we know about them? The state of the evidence of programs, costs and impacts on health outcomes of using community health workers. *World Health Organization, Geneva.*

McPherson, M., Smith-Lovin, L., & Cook, J. M. (2001). Birds of a feather: Homophily in social networks. *Annual Review of Sociology, 27*, 415–444.

Mutchler, M. G., & McDavitt, B. (2011). 'Gay boy talk' meets 'girl talk': HIV risk assessment assumptions in young gay men's sexual health communication with best friends. *Health Education Research, 26*(3), 489–505. https://doi.org/10.1093/her/cyq069

O'Brien, M. J., Squires, A. P., Bixby, R. A., & Larson, S. C. (2009). Role development of community health workers: An examination of selection and training processes in the intervention literature. *American Journal of Preventive Medicine, 37*(6, Supplement 1), S262–S269. https://doi.org/10.1016/j.amepre.2009.08.011

O'Connor, M., Sanson, A., Hawkins, M. T., Letcher, P., Toumbourou, J. W., Smart, D., Vassallo, S., & Olsson, C. A. (2011). Predictors of positive development in emerging adulthood. *Journal of Youth and Adolescence, 40*(7), 860–874. https://doi.org/10.1007/s10964-010-9593-7

Olaniran, A., Smith, H., Unkels, R., Bar-Zeev, S., & van den Broek, N. (2017). Who is a community health worker? – A systematic review of definitions. *Global Health Action, 10*(1), 1272223. https://doi.org/10.1080/16549716.2017.1272223

Olaniran, A., Madaj, B., Bar-Zev, S., & van den Broek, N. (2019). The roles of community health workers who provide maternal and newborn health services: Case studies from Africa and Asia. *BMJ Global Health, 4*(4), e001388. https://doi.org/10.1136/bmjgh-2019-001388

Pérez, L. M., & Martinez, J. (2008). Community health workers: social justice and policy advocates for community health and well-being. *American Journal of Public Health, 98*(1), 11–14.

Phillips, G., McCuskey, D., Ruprecht, M. M., Curry, C. W., & Felt, D. (2021). Structural interventions for HIV prevention and care among US men who have sex with men: A systematic review of evidence, gaps, and future priorities. *AIDS and Behavior., 25*, 2907–2919. https://doi.org/10.1007/s10461-021-03167-2

Pichon, L. C., Teti, M., McGoy, S., Murry, V. M., & Juarez, P. D. (2022). Engaging Black men who have sex with men (MSM) in the South in identifying strategies to increase PrEP uptake. *BMC Health Services Research, 22*(1), 1491. https://doi.org/10.1186/s12913-022-08914-2

Quinn, K., Dickson-Gomez, J., Zarwell, M., Pearson, B., & Lewis, M. (2018). "A gay man and a doctor are just like, a recipe for destruction": How racism and homonegativity in healthcare settings influence PrEP uptake among young Black MSM. *AIDS and Behavior., 23*, 1951–1963. https://doi.org/10.1007/s10461-018-2375-z

Quinn, K. G., Christenson, E., Spector, A., Amirkhanian, Y., & Kelly, J. A. (2020). The influence of peers on PrEP perceptions and use among young Black gay, bisexual, and other men who have sex with men: A qualitative examination. *Archives of Sexual Behavior., 49*, 2129–2143. https://doi.org/10.1007/s10508-019-01593-x

Schneider, J. A., Zhou, A. N., & Laumann, E. O. (2015). A new HIV prevention network approach: Sociometric peer change agent selection. *Social Science & Medicine, 125*(Supplement C), 192–202. https://doi.org/10.1016/j.socscimed.2013.12.034

Simoni, J. M., Nelson, K. M., Franks, J. C., Yard, S. S., & Lehavot, K. (2011). Are peer interventions for HIV efficacious? A systematic review. *AIDS and Behavior, 15*(8), 1589–1595. https://doi.org/10.1007/s10461-011-9963-5

Steinberg, L., & Morris, A. S. (2001). Adolescent development. *Annual Review of Psychology, 52*, 83–110. https://doi.org/10.1146/annurev.psych.52.1.83

Street, R. L., & Gordon, H. S. (2008). Companion participation in cancer consultations. *Psycho-Oncology, 17*(3), 244–251. https://doi.org/10.1002/pon.1225

Viswanathan, M., Kraschnewski, J. L., Nishikawa, B., Morgan, L. C., Honeycutt, A. A., Thieda, P., Lohr, K. N., & Jonas, D. E. (2010). Outcomes and costs of community health worker interventions: A systematic review. *Medical Care, 48*(9), 792–808. https://doi.org/10.1097/MLR.0b013e3181e35b51

Weeks, M. R., Convey, M., Dickson-Gomez, J., Li, J., Radda, K., Martinez, M., & Robles, E. (2009). Changing drug users' risk environments: Peer health advocates as multi-level community change agents. *American Journal of Community Psychology, 43*(3), 330–344. https://doi.org/10.1007/s10464-009-9234-z

White, J. J., Yang, C., Tobin, K. E., Beyrer, C., & Latkin, C. A. (2020). Individual and social network factors associated with high self-efficacy of communicating about men's health issues with peers among Black MSM in an urban setting. *Journal of Urban Health, 97*(5), 668–678. https://doi.org/10.1007/s11524-020-00458-2

World Health Organization. (2018). *WHO guideline on health policy and system support to optimize community health worker programmes*. World Health Organization. https://iris.who.int/handle/10665/275474

Young, L. E., Schumm, P., Alon, L., Bouris, A., Ferreira, M., Hill, B., Khanna, A. S., Valente, T. W., & Schneider, J. A. (2017). PrEP Chicago: A randomized controlled peer change agent intervention to promote the adoption of pre-exposure prophylaxis for HIV prevention among young Black men who have sex with men. *Clinical Trials, 1740774517730012*, 44–52. https://doi.org/10.1177/1740774517730012

Olaniran, A., Smith, H., Unkels, R., Bar-Zeev, S., & van den Broek, N. (2017). Who is a community health worker? – A systematic review of definitions. *Global Health Action, 10*(1), 1272223. https://doi.org/10.1080/16549716.2017.1272223

Olaniran, A., Madaj, B., Bar-Zev, S., & van den Broek, N. (2019). The roles of community health workers who provide maternal and newborn health services: Case studies from Africa and Asia. *BMJ Global Health, 4*(4), e001388. https://doi.org/10.1136/bmjgh-2019-001388

Perez, L. M., & Martinez, J. (2008). Community health workers: Social justice and policy advocates for community health and well-being. *American Journal of Public Health, 98*(1), 11–14.

Phillips, G., McCuskey, D., Ruprecht, M. M., Curry, C. W., & Felt, D. (2021). Structural interventions for HIV prevention and care among US men who have sex with men: A systematic review of evidence, gaps, and future priorities. *AIDS and Behavior, 25*, 2907–2919. https://doi.org/10.1007/s10461-021-03167-2

Pichon, L. C., Teti, M., McGoy, S., Murry, V. M., & Juarez, P. D. (2022). Engaging Black men who have sex with men (MSM) in the South in identifying strategies to increase PrEP uptake. *BMC Health Services Research, 22*(1), 1491. https://doi.org/10.1186/s12913-022-08874-3

Quinn, K., Dickson-Gomez, J., Zarwell, M., Pearson, B., & Lewis, M. (2018). "A gay man and a doctor are just like, a recipe for destruction": How racism and homonegativity in healthcare settings influence PrEP uptake among young Black MSM. *AIDS and Behavior, 23*, 1951–1963. https://doi.org/10.1007/s10461-018-2375-z

Quinn, K. G., Christenson, E., Spector, A., Amirkhanian, Y., & Kelly, J. A. (2020). The influence of peers on PrEP perceptions and use among young Black gay, bisexual, and other men who have sex with men: A qualitative examination. *Archives of Sexual Behavior, 49*, 2129–2143. https://doi.org/10.1007/s10508-019-01593-x

Schneider, J. A., Zhou, A. N., & Laumann, E. O. (2015). A new HIV prevention network approach: Sociometric peer change agent selection. *Social Science & Medicine, 125*(Supplement C), 192–202. https://doi.org/10.1016/j.socscimed.2013.12.034

Simoni, J. M., Nelson, K. M., Franks, J. C., Yard, S. S., & Lehavot, K. (2011). Are peer interventions for HIV efficacious? A systematic review. *AIDS and Behavior, 15*(8), 1589–1595. https://doi.org/10.1007/s10461-011-9963-5

Steinberg, L., & Morris, A. S. (2001). Adolescent development. *Annual Review of Psychology, 52*, 83–110. https://doi.org/10.1146/annurev.psych.52.1.83

Street, R. L., & Gordon, H. S. (2008). Companion participation in cancer consultations. *Psycho-Oncology, 17*(3), 244–251. https://doi.org/10.1002/pon.1225

Viswanathan, M., Kraschnewski, J. L., Nishikawa, B., Morgan, L. C., Honeycutt, A. A., Thieda, P., Lohr, K. N., & Jonas, D. E. (2010). Outcomes and costs of community health worker interventions: A systematic review. *Medical Care, 48*(9), 792–808. https://doi.org/10.1097/MLR.0b013e3181e35b51

Weeks, M. R., Convey, M., Dickson-Gomez, J., Li, J., Radda, K., Martinez, M., & Robles, E. (2009). Changing drug users' risk environments: Peer health advocates as multi-level community change agents. *American Journal of Community Psychology, 43*(3), 330–344. https://doi.org/10.1007/s10464-009-9234-z

White, J. J., Yang, C., Tobin, K. E., Beyrer, C., & Latkin, C. A. (2020). Individual and social network factors associated with high self-efficacy of communicating about men's health issues with peers among Black MSM in an urban setting. *Journal of Urban Health, 97*(5), 668–678. https://doi.org/10.1007/s11524-020-00458-2

World Health Organization. (2018). *WHO guideline on health policy and system support to optimize community health worker programmes*. World Health Organization. https://iris.who.int/handle/10665/275474

Young, L. E., Schumm, P., Alon, L., Bouris, A., Ferreira, M., Hill, B., Khanna, A. S., Valente, T. W., & Schneider, J. A. (2018). PrEP Chicago: A randomized controlled peer change agent intervention to promote the adoption of pre-exposure prophylaxis for HIV prevention among young Black men who have sex with men. *Clinical Trials, 15*(1), 44–52. https://doi.org/10.1177/1740774517730012

Chapter 7
Tailored and Targeted Health Communication

Chapter Objectives

1. Describe the personalization continuum in health communication.
2. Analyze the differences between tailored and targeted communication strategies.
3. Evaluate the effectiveness of tailored and targeted health communication strategies.

The Personalization Continuum in Health Communication

The personalization continuum refers to the range of health communication and other intervention approaches that are used to address individual patient characteristics, preferences, and needs (Fig. 7.1). It reflects a shift from a one-size-fits-all public health communication model to a more person-centered approach (as discussed in Chap. 4), promoting greater health outcomes and patient satisfaction (Tutton, 2012). On one end of the spectrum is a broad approach that is used for the general population (e.g., a general condom use campaign for safe sex), where prevention scientists and public health practitioners design mass media campaigns based on general population data and standardized protocols. Moving along the continuum, health communication messages and intervention approaches incorporate more specific information such as demographic characteristics, lifestyle, and personal values to become increasingly customized for the target group. At the far end of the other side of the continuum lies personalized medicine, which uses innovative technologies such as machine learning to design highly individualized treatment plans (Wray et al., 2019). The progression along the personalization continuum enhances the relevance (and therefore the effectiveness) of health communication and intervention strategies by aligning more closely with individual profiles

D. T. Dangerfield II, *Prevention Science & Targeted Methods for HIV/STI Research with Black Sexual Minority Men*,
https://doi.org/10.1007/978-3-031-85130-8_7

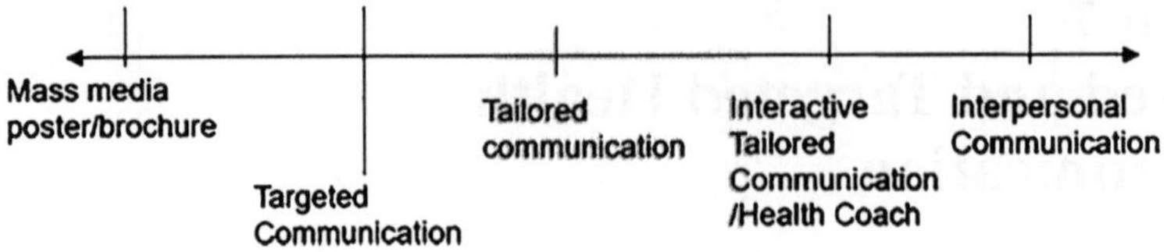

Fig. 7.1 Personalization continuum of health communication

(Schleidgen et al., 2013). Ultimately, the continuum underscores the importance of tailored and targeted communication in meaningful engagement with diverse populations and maximizing the impact of health interventions.

What Is Targeted Health Communication?

Targeted health communication refers to the intentional design and delivery of prevention messages (or interventions) to specific population subgroups based on characteristics such as age, gender, ethnicity, health status, or behavior (Kreuter & Wray, 2003). Targeted interventions leverage research findings to adapt or modify content in a way that resonates more effectively with the specific subpopulation to enhance its impact. For example, targeted HIV/STI prevention programs that consider the specific motivations and barriers experienced by Black SMM would focus on the specific facilitators and barriers to prevention behaviors of that community relative to the general population (Dangerfield II et al., 2022; Elion et al., 2019; Krueger & Casey, 2014). Targeted interventions within the broad community of sexual minorities might also focus on the specific needs of Black SMM relative to the general LGBTQ+ community. Targeted interventions and health communication programs increase awareness, influence attitudes, and promote health behaviors by addressing the unique needs, preferences, and cultural contexts of population subgroups (Elion et al., 2019; Jones et al., 2008; Wilton et al., 2009). Ultimately, targeted health interventions seek to improve public health by ensuring that important health information is accessible, understandable, and actionable for population subgroups (Noar et al., 2007).

Building the Case for Targeted Strategies

Research shows that targeted messaging not only enhances the relevance and impact of the information but also builds trust and credibility within these communities, leading to increased uptake of prevention strategies and reducing disease incidence (Elion et al., 2019; Habarta et al., 2017). Targeted sexual health messaging for Black

SMM is essential due to the disproportionate impact of HIV on the community. Remember in Chap. 1 that Black SMM have experienced the greatest disparities in HIV/STI incidence and outcomes for two decades. These disparities are driven by a combination of individual, social, economic, and structural factors (including sexual epidemiology [see Chap. 1]) that affects them differently than others. By targeting prevention and treatment messages to address the unique cultural, social, and behavioral contexts of the community, public health interventions can more effectively increase knowledge and prevention behaviors, including PrEP. Culturally specific campaigns can address the unique barriers these men face such as medical mistrust and anticipated discrimination by providing relatable, affirming, and stigma-free information. Targeted messages are essential even when innovations are expected to diffuse theoretically because the process of diffusion is not uniform across all segments of the population. Targeted sexual health efforts can make significant strides in reducing subgroup differences in public health outcomes by acknowledging and addressing the specific needs of Black SMM. Targeted messages are crucial for ensuring that all population segments benefit from the innovation. By designing culturally relevant and sensitive messages, public health initiatives can more effectively engage these communities, foster trust, and encourage uptake.

Moreover, targeting subgroups for prevention and treatment activities is more effective and economical than intervening on everyone, including targeting all Black SMM. For example, a modeling study showed that targeting PrEP to 20% of the highest risk HIV-negative SMM could prevent twice as many infections over 20 years and at better economic value than providing PrEP to 20% of all HIV-negative sexual minority men (Juusola et al., 2012). Data show that avoiding one HIV infection could save $229,800 and reduced U.S. incidence by ~70% by 2025 if targeted intervention strategies increased linkage to care (Juusola et al., 2012; Marshall et al., 2018). The treatment costs of individuals living with HIV is expensive for the healthcare system because (at this point) patients need medical care across for the rest of their lifespan. Preventing HIV and STIs among Black SMM therefore has a dual savings benefit given symbiotic relationship between infections. High-risk care management models reduce costs and improve health by targeting a proportion of highest risk patients using evidence-based strategies. Therefore, investing in targeted prevention and intervention efforts for Black SMM not only addresses significant health disparities but also provides substantial economic benefits by reducing the long-term financial burden on the healthcare system.

Using Theory to Help Build the Case for Targeted Interventions

Behavior change theories can also help build the case for targeted intervention approaches. For example, Diffusion of Innovations theory posits that new interventions will follow a predictable pattern of uptake across different segments of the population because individuals adopt new behaviors when they see "early adopters" successfully using them (Rogers & Adhikarya, 1979; Schuyler et al., 2021). According to this theory, as new prevention regimens such as PrEP becomes more widely accepted and visible within key communities, it will gradually diffuse through the population, encouraging broader acceptance and use (Hosek, 2013; Schuyler et al., 2021; Young et al., 2017). Theoretically, targeted messages can help to address these differences by adapting communication strategies to the specific needs, barriers, and motivators of each group. Theoretically, innovators and early adopters, who are typically more open to new ideas and have greater access to information and healthcare resources, would be the first in the community to use PrEP. These individuals are often opinion leaders within their communities and play a crucial role in influencing subsequent adoption. As they demonstrate the benefits and effectiveness of PrEP, the early majority, who are more deliberate but still receptive to new innovations, will begin to adopt the practice. Following them, the late majority, who may be more skeptical and require more evidence and reassurance, will start to use PrEP as it becomes more widely accepted and normalized. Finally, the laggards, who are the most resistant to change and often have the least access to healthcare resources, will theoretically adopt PrEP last. This phased approach highlights the importance of targeted education, outreach, and support programs at each stage to address specific barriers and facilitators of PrEP adoption (Rogers & Adhikarya, 1979; Schuyler et al., 2021). Although theory provides a framework for understanding how innovations spread, targeted messages are necessary to facilitate and accelerate this process, ensuring that all groups, particularly those at higher risk or with greater barriers, can benefit from the innovation (Dangerfield II et al., 2021; Kreuter & Wray, 2003; Rogers et al., 2019).

Targeted HIV Prevention Campaigns for Black Sexual Minority Men

Targeted sexual health campaigns are crucial for addressing the unique health disparities and challenges experienced Black SMM. By incorporating community insights (especially from "targeted" studies) and collaborating with local leaders, these targeted initiative provide relevant information about HIV prevention and treatment options in ways that resonate specifically with the community. For example, the "Testing Makes Us Stronger" campaign was an innovative and effective public health campaign specifically targeting Black gay and bisexual men to promote regular HIV testing (Habarta et al., 2017). Launched by the Centers for Disease Control and Prevention (CDC) in 2011, the campaign aimed to reduce HIV-related stigma and empower Black gay and bisexual men by emphasizing the strength and resilience in knowing their HIV status. The campaign featured positive representations of Black gay men and included culturally relevant messages that fostered a sense of pride and community. The "Testing Makes Us Stronger" campaign leveraged social media, online platforms, and community-based events to reach Black gay men where they were to make HIV testing less intimidating. "Testing Makes Us Stronger" successfully encouraged more frequent testing and opened up critical dialogues about HIV prevention and care by highlighting personal stories and providing clear information on where and how to get tested. The campaign's focus on empowerment and health equity helped to address the disproportionate impact of HIV on Black gay men and contributed to broader efforts to reduce health disparities in this population (Boudewyns et al., 2018; Habarta et al., 2017). Therefore, this targeted campaign successfully increased HIV testing among Black gay and bisexual men, leading to greater awareness and early detection of HIV among this vulnerable community. As a result, this health communication initiative provided crucial information as well as empowerment, destigmatization, and informed decision-making for Black gay and bisexual men. Moreover, this targeted sexual health campaign created a supportive environment where Black gay men could make informed health decisions and access resources without judgment or marginalization.

Designing Targeted Health Communication Messages

Designing targeted health communication messages involves several key steps to ensure that the information resonates with specific subpopulations and effectively influences their health behaviors (Kreuter & Wray, 2003). By following these steps, health communication messages can be effectively targeted to meet the specific needs and preferences of different population segments, thereby enhancing their impact and contributing to better health outcomes (Kreuter & Wray, 2003; Noar et al., 2007, 2009).

1. **Identify and understand the target subpopulation.** Divide the community into a smaller, more homogenous groups based on characteristics such as age, gender, ethnicity, health status, or even behavior. Then study the characteristics and needs of that group using surveys, in-depth qualitative interviews, focus groups, and/or existing data to better understand their attitudes, beliefs, cultural norms, and health behaviors.
2. **Engage and collaborate with community leaders.** Collaborate with trusted community leaders and organizations to co-create and disseminate messages (see Chap. 3). Their endorsement can enhance credibility and acceptance. Establish ways to receive feedback from the community to refine and improve the messages continuously.
3. **Define clear intervention objectives.** Determine what the intervention plans to achieve. Does it involve increasing awareness, changing behavior, or promoting the use of novel treatments? Establish measures and metrics to assess the effectiveness of the intervention or health communication campaign, such as the number of people who are tested for HIV or use PrEP.
4. **Create culturally relevant and appropriate content.** Ensure that the message respects and incorporates the cultural values and norms of the target audience.

Use language, images, and examples that the community can relate to. This might involve testimonials from community members or culturally relevant metaphors and/or analogies. Culturally relevant messaging should be designed in collaboration with the target population.

5. **Use appropriate dissemination channels and formats.** Identify media preferences and choose communication channels that the target audience frequently uses, such as social media, or healthcare provider networks. Multiple dissemination mechanisms such as videos, infographics, brochures, and interactive web tools can cater to different preferences and literacy levels.
6. **Test and refine messages.** Conduct pilot tests of the messages with a small segment of the target audience to gauge their reactions and understanding. Use the feedback from pre-testing to modify and improve the messages before a broader rollout.
7. **Monitor and evaluate the campaign.** Continuously monitor the campaign's reach and impact using surveys, focus groups, and/or health outcome data. Be prepared to adjust the communication strategies based on what is working and what is not to ensure the messages remain effective and relevant.

The Role of Culture on Message Design and Effectiveness

Culture substantially influences the effectiveness of health messages by shaping individuals' beliefs, values, behaviors, and perceptions regarding health and illness (Aggleton et al., 2015; Airhihenbuwa et al., 2014; Kreuter et al., 2003). Understanding the cultural context of the target audience enables prevention scientists to craft messages that resonate more deeply, are more likely to be accepted, and more likely to be acted upon. Cultural competence involves understanding and acknowledging the diverse backgrounds, languages, and traditions of different groups. Addressing cultural stigmas and norms surrounding health issues, such as sexuality, mental health, or sexual health, can help overcome communication barriers and promote more open, effective dialogues (Hosek et al., 2015).

For Black SMM, Black and gay culture plays a crucial role in shaping health beliefs, behaviors, and attitudes toward healthcare. For example, cultural experiences of discrimination based on race or sexuality in society and clinical settings have led to mistrust of medical institutions and reluctance generally to seek prevention and treatment services despite interest in their own health maintenance (Arnold et al., 2014; Quinn et al., 2018). This can also impact their reception of sexual health messages from the medical community. Additionally, nuanced regarding sexuality impact perceptions of risk and prevention needs assessments (See Chap. 1 on Sexual Epidemiology). Effective health communication for this group requires incorporating cultural competence and sensitivity, acknowledging the unique challenges they face. Using culturally relevant language, symbols, and narratives that reflect their lived experiences can enhance relatability and trust. Designing health messages with the cultural realities of Black gay men in mind can foster greater trust, engagement, and ultimately, better health outcomes. Culturally specific health messages are not only more respectful and inclusive but significantly more effective in driving positive health behaviors and outcomes (Hosek et al., 2015).

Advantages and Disadvantages of Targeted Health Messages and Interventions

Targeted sexual health messages and interventions offer significant advantages, particularly in their ability to more effectively resonate with specific population using language, symbols, and narratives that are familiar and relevant to target audiences to address their unique cultural, social, and behavioral contexts. Targeted strategies can also build trust and credibility, especially when disseminated through popular community leaders and culturally appropriate channels. However, there are also disadvantages to consider. First, targeted messages may inadvertently exclude or overlook subgroups within the broader target population, potentially leading to additional feelings of marginalization or neglect, especially among racial and sexual minority men who often have background feelings of exclusion. There is also a risk of reinforcing stereotypes if the messages are not carefully designed with community input, which can result in backlash or reduced effectiveness (Calabrese et al., 2023). Designing and implementing targeted interventions can also be time- and labor-intensive because they require extensive research and collaboration to ensure cultural relevance. Balancing specificity with inclusivity and maintaining sensitivity to the diverse experiences within a target group is crucial in the design of effective targeted sexual health messages.

Acknowledging Subgroup Differences

Even within subgroups that are based upon similar characteristics, everyone is not the same. Acknowledging differences within subpopulations is as crucial in designing effective health communication strategies as targeting to the entire subgroup because diversity within populations also means that health behaviors, beliefs, and access to resources vary. These within-group differences can also affect how health messages are received and acted upon in the community. Black gay and bisexual men have different cultural norms, levels of health literacy, and health behaviors (Dangerfield II et al., 2018, 2021). Targeting health communication and interventions to address these unique characteristics ensures that treatments are relevant, understandable, and persuasive for each subgroup. Prevention scientists can further overcome barriers to effective communication, build trust within communities, and ultimately improve the overall health and well-being of diverse populations by customizing messages to align with the specific needs and contexts of different subgroups within target populations (Noar et al., 2007).

Applying Person Centered Approaches to Identify and Target Subgroups for HIV Prevention Messaging

Chapter 4 identified the usefulness of person-centered statistical approaches for targeted intervention design. The current guidelines for PrEP can be used to reinforce the application of person centered approaches and targeted intervention design. For example, the CDC recommends PrEP use for HIV-negative adult men who have sex with men who report any of the following criteria: (1) any male partner in the past 6 months; (2) not in a monogamous partnership with another HIV-uninfected man and; (3) condomless anal sex or an STI in the past 6 months (Centers for Disease Control and Prevention, 2018). Additional sexual risk indicators include drug use and being in a sexual relationship with HIV seropositive male partners. However, as discussed in Chaps. 1 and 2, Black gay and bisexual men are less likely to meet CDC PrEP indicators than other racial/ethnic groups despite having an acute risk for HIV acquisition (Ezennia et al., 2019; Lancki et al., 2018; Rolle et al., 2017). Studies show that only 52–65% of Black SMM who seroconverted had an indication for PrEP based on CDC guidelines (Hoots et al., 2016; Lancki et al., 2018; Sullivan et al., 2015). This suggests that evaluating sexual risk among Black gay and bisexual men requires more targeted approaches to identify best PrEP candidates.

I led a latent class analysis to examine the profiles of sexual risk and PrEP use patterns among Black SMM in the HPTN 073 Study based upon CDC guidelines (Dangerfield II et al., 2021), which we discussed in Chap. 4. We identified three distinct subgroups of Black gay and bisexual men: "Single with Condomless Partners," "Single with Multiple Partners," and "Serodiscordant Partners." Single with Condomless Partners comprised most of the sample (69.4%), followed by Single, Multiple Partners (19.0%), then Serodiscordant Partners (11.5%). Different messaging strategies could be used to target Black SMM of different risk profiles. Potentially, a clinical tool could be designed to classify and identify the relative sexual risk and PrEP need of individuals with multiple risk indicators. Future research should continue to identify profiles of sexual risk generally and among Black SMM and test targeted strategies among population subgroups.

Tailored Communication and Intervention Approaches

Tailored interventions are customized strategies designed to address the specific needs, characteristics, and circumstances of individuals or target groups (Kreuter & Wray, 2003; Noar et al., 2007). These interventions are designed based on detailed assessments and data collection, ensuring they are relevant and effective for the intended audience. Tailored interventions aim to enhance engagement, compliance, and overall outcomes by considering factors such as cultural background, personal preferences, health status, and environmental context for more personalized approach along the continuum. Evidence for tailoring interventions highlights several key benefits. First, tailored interventions are more relevant to individuals, making them more likely to be read and remembered. They are perceived as having higher personal relevance, which enhances their effectiveness. Research shows that tailored health communication strategies can lead to better health outcomes by increasing engagement, enhancing comprehension, and promoting behavior change more effectively than one-size-fits-all approaches (Bauermeister et al., 2015; Wanyonyi et al., 2011). This approach leads to higher perceived risk and motivation to change, as well as greater self-efficacy (Bauermeister et al., 2015). Consequently, tailored interventions often result in more significant behavior changes compared to generic approaches (Wanyonyi et al., 2011). This personalized approach contrasts with one-size-fits-all solutions, offering a more nuanced and potentially more successful pathway to achieving desired results in health education and behavior change. Therefore, tailored interventions represent a much needed and effective strategy in prevention science approach, particularly for addressing complex health behaviors and disparities within diverse populations.

Motivational Interviewing for Tailored Communication

Motivational interviewing (MI) is a widely used tailored communication approach that can activate sexual health behavior change (Miller & Rollnick, 2012; Rollnick & Miller, 1995). MI collaborates with a client (or patient) to activate their motivations to change behavior using open-ended interviewing and reflective listening (Rollnick & Miller, 1995). This tailored communication strategy has been shown to improve patient engagement, adherence to treatment plans, and overall health outcomes (Miller & Rollnick, 2009). Studies have demonstrated that MI can significantly increase the uptake of PrEP and enhance engagement in regular HIV testing and safer sexual practices among high-risk populations, including Black SMM (Miller & Rollnick, 2012; Dangerfield II et al., 2023). Some HIV prevention interventions utilize "MI consistent" or "MI-based" interviews to improve PrEP willingness and use because of their cost-effectiveness, brevity, and utilization of client interests for behavior change (Dangerfield II et al., 2023; Moitra et al., 2020; Psaros et al., 2014). However, existing MI-based interventions to improve PrEP are limited because of methodological inconsistencies (e.g., credentials of MI counselors, theoretical guidance, session content, duration of session, study protocol) and even further limited among Black SMM (Dangerfield II et al., 2023).

POSSIBLE as a Tailored and Targeted Sexual Health Intervention

Chapter 6 discussed how POSSIBLE used a peer change agent (PCA) to improve HIV risk perceptions and PrEP use among Black SMM. POSSIBLE leveraged MI as a tailored health intervention for Black gay men by integrating it into scripted conversations that addressed participants' lifestyles, personal goals, and HIV risks facilitated by a PrEP-using PCA. The script allowed the PCA to discuss a participant's lifestyles, personal goals and values, relative HIV risks, and PRH with everyone in similar ways but also tailor messages based upon the responses of specific individuals (Dangerfield II & Anderson, 2024). Example questions included, "*How would being diagnosed with HIV impact your goals*?" and "*What do you think about your HIV risk given that estimates suggest that 50% of Black SMM will acquire it*?" The script also provided opportunities for the PCA to address HIV/PrEP misinformation and disclose PrEP use to share experiences managing potential side effects, challenges disclosing use to romantic/sexual partners, and empathy regarding participants' stigmatizing clinical experiences (Dangerfield II, 2023). The scripted conversations were designed to capture the "spirit of MI" (Miller & Rollnick, 2012; Rollnick et al., 2010) while guiding participants to realize their HIV vulnerability and move along the stages of change to consider PrEP use. Specifically, the script allows the PCA to gather information about the participant and target opportunities to share personal information that might catalyze their interest in PrEP or change their attitudes toward their PRH. Towards the end of the session, the script guides the PCA to tailor prevention messaging to influence PHR and encourage PrEP use regardless of participants' reported behaviors. The script provides a guide for the PCA's tailored responses based upon what participants say about their goals, values, and behaviors to try to catalyze changes in PHR and PrEP regardless of behavior. For example, if a participant expressed concern about potential side effects of PrEP, the PCA might share their own experiences with managing those side effects, emphasizing how PrEP use aligns with the participant's personal goals of staying healthy and protecting their future. Similarly, if a participant downplayed their HIV risk due to a lack of perceived vulnerability, the PCA could gently challenge this perception by highlighting the high statistical risk for Black SMM and framing PrEP as a proactive step toward safeguarding their health and achieving their life goals. I published data demonstrating these findings in the *Journal of Environmental Research and Public Health* in an autoethnography (Dangerfield II, 2023):

Participant (Age 26): I don't think I need PrEP because I'm in a relationship.

Peer Change Agent: *Are y'all using condoms?*

Participant: No. We are monogamous though.

Peer Change Agent: *I totally get it. That's something that I struggle with myself. I saw some research from Atlanta a while ago suggesting that most people who were newly infected with HIV acquired it from people they considered "main partners." I have my thoughts about what it means to be a main partner, but as Black gay men we really can't afford to take any chances with our health. Since you said you don't want HIV, I think you should still use it because we just never know what someone else is doing and I care about your health. What do you think?*

Participant: Wow. I think you're right. You really never know.

In alignment with the "spirit of MI" (Miller & Rollnick, 2012; Rollnick & Miller, 1995) the scripted PCA builds rapport, engages participants, actively listens, and evokes intrinsic motivations while expanding upon MI by gently encouraging PrEP use within the context of their lives. In this example, this person was willing to be referred to PrEP for HIV prevention. Potentially, this adapted model of MI requires further study and validation, as it assumes that individuals are open to considering

PrEP in the first place, while MI's core principle is to draw out behaviors that individuals themselves identify as priorities for change. This approach not only helped identify of ambivalence and barriers but also enabled the PCA to guide participants towards a (research-driven) desired beahavior using personalized messages at the end of every interview. Baseline results showed a statistically significant improvement in PRH after the one 20-minute session (Dangerfield II & Anderson, 2024). Additionally, 64% were willing to be referred to PrEP care after baseline; 45% of whom made a PrEP appointment. PRH was not associated with referral willingness.

POSSIBLE demonstrates the potential for targeted interventions to enhance engagement and improve health outcomes in marginalized communities using scripted yet tailored communication responses to motivate behavior change. Overall, POSSIBLE exemplifies how a theoretically guided, culturally competent health communication intervention can effectively target the unique needs and of Black SMM and tailor prevention messages to improve health behaviors. This approach ensures that each conversation remains rooted in the participant's reality while subtly steering them toward behavior change, aligning with the spirit of MI to foster self-reflection, autonomy, and informed decision-making about their sexual health (Miller & Rollnick, 2012). The data published from these sessions not only demonstrated the effectiveness of this tailored intervention but also provided insights into how personalized conversations can be leveraged to address complex health behaviors in marginalized communities, ultimately contributing to the broader discourse on HIV prevention and health equity.

Advantages and Disadvantages of Tailoring Health Communication and Interventions

Tailored health communication interventions offer significant advantages because they allow prevention scientists to customize messages that align with the specific characteristics, needs, and preferences of individuals or subgroups, which enhances treatment relevance, engagement, and effectiveness (Kreuter et al., 2000; Noar et al., 2007). Tailored approaches can lead to higher rates of behavior change, improved health outcomes, and greater patient satisfaction (Kreuter et al., 2000; Noar et al., 2007). However, designing tailored interventions is resource-intensive, requires extensive data collection and sophisticated analyses to create personalized content. Additionally, since tailored messages are different for everyone, it may be difficult to pinpoint exactly how and which messages in health communication have the impact on the individual, which could be difficult to replicate (Beck et al., 2010). Tailored messages could also inadvertently exclude or overlook some individuals within the broader target population, potentially leading to feelings of marginalization. Balancing the benefits of specificity with broad applicability and ensuring inclusivity remain challenges in the implementation of tailored health communication interventions.

Using Novel Technologies for Tailored Interventions

New technology can be leveraged to design tailored interventions through several innovative approaches. First, data analytics and machine learning algorithms can process large datasets to identify patterns and personalize interventions based on individual behaviors, preferences, and needs (Wray et al., 2019). Wearable devices and mobile apps can continuously monitor health metrics, providing real-time feedback and personalized recommendations. Additionally, AI can enhance the personalization of content by dynamically adjusting messages and interventions based on user interactions and progress. Virtual reality and augmented reality can also create immersive experiences that adapt to the user's specific context and learning style, enhancing engagement and effectiveness. Moreover, telehealth platforms enable remote and individualized support from professionals, making tailored interventions more accessible and scalable. Together, these technologies provide powerful tools to create more precise, effective, and engaging interventions tailored to individual needs.

Conclusion

Targeted and tailored interventions are essential for addressing the specific health needs of minority communities. These interventions are crucial for advancing public health equity, improving health outcomes, and reducing disparities. Integrating theoretical frameworks and novel technologies can further enhance the effectiveness of these tailored strategies. Targeted and tailored interventions for sexual health promotion are crucial for sexual minority communities due to their unique and specific health needs that are often overlooked by general health programs. These interventions recognize the diverse experiences and challenges faced by sexual minorities, such as stigma, discrimination, and higher risks of infectious diseases. These interventions can effectively address barriers to healthcare access, promote safer sexual practices, and enhance the uptake of preventive measures like PrEP. Moreover, tailored interventions foster trust and engagement within these communities, leading to better health outcomes and reduced health disparities. Ensuring that sexual health promotion is inclusive and responsive to the needs of Black SMM is essential for advancing public health equity.

Raised Questions

1. What communication domains should be considered when designing targeted and tailored sexual health messages, especially for population subgroups?

2. Which theoretical frameworks can best enhance the effectiveness of targeted and tailored health messages for Black SMM?
3. What strategies can help scale the delivery of tailored health communication strategies effectively and ethically for the community?

Chapter Summary

This chapter focused on the significance of personalized health communication strategies, particularly in addressing the unique needs of various population subgroups. It outlined the "personalization continuum," which ranges from broad, general public health messages to highly individualized interventions using advanced technologies like machine learning. Then the chapter emphasized that targeted and tailored health communication can enhance the effectiveness of public health interventions by aligning them more closely with the specific characteristics, preferences, and needs of individuals or subpopulations. Several strategies and examples were provided to demonstrate the effectiveness and promise of targeted and tailored sexual health communication approaches among Black SMM.

Key Points

1. **Targeted health communication**: Targeted health communication focuses on designing messages for specific subpopulations by considering their unique demographic, cultural, and behavioral contexts. Targeted strategies are more effective in increasing awareness, influencing attitudes, and promoting health behaviors within communities.
2. **Cultural relevance in health communication**: The role of culture in health communication is crucial. Culturally competent messaging that acknowledges the specific challenges and experiences in communities, enhances engagement, and promotes better health outcomes. Effective health communication must be culturally sensitive and respectful to resonate with the target audience.
3. **Acknowledging subgroup differences**. Not everyone in a population (or subpopulation) is the same. Therefore, health campaigns should account for these variations by tailoring messages, strategies, and interventions to align with the unique cultural, demographic, behavioral, and psychosocial characteristics of different subgroups.
4. **Tailored health communication and motivational interviewing (MI)**: Tailored health communication customizes messages to an individual's specific characteristics, needs, and circumstances. Motivational interviewing (MI) is highlighted as a tailored communication strategy that uses personalized dialogue to encourage behavior change, such as PrEP uptake. Tailored interventions have

been shown to improve health behaviors by making messages more personally relevant and impactful.

5. **Advantages and challenges of tailored communication**: Tailored health interventions are more relevant and effective than general messages. However, designing these interventions is resource-intensive and can be challenging to scale. Balancing specificity with inclusivity and ensuring that tailored messages do not inadvertently exclude individuals within the target population is a key challenge in their implementation.

References

Aggleton, P., Parker, R., & Thomas, F. (2015). Sexuality, culture, and society: Shifting paradigms in sexuality research. In *Culture, health and sexuality: An introduction* (pp. 251–266). Routledge.

Airhihenbuwa, C. O., Ford, C. L., & Iwelunmor, J. I. (2014). Why culture matters in health interventions: Lessons from HIV/AIDS stigma and NCDs. *Health Education & Behavior, 41*(1), 78–84. https://doi.org/10.1177/1090198113487199

Arnold, E. A., Rebchook, G. M., & Kegeles, S. M. (2014). "Triply cursed": Racism, homophobia, and HIV-related stigma are barriers to regular HIV testing, treatment adherence, and disclosure among young Black gay men. *Culture, Health & Sexuality, 16*(6), 710–722. https://doi.org/10.1080/13691058.2014.905706

Bauermeister, J. A., Pingel, E. S., Jadwin-Cakmak, L., Harper, G. W., Horvath, K., Weiss, G., & Dittus, P. (2015). Acceptability and preliminary efficacy of a tailored online HIV/STI testing intervention for young men who have sex with men: The get connected! Program. *AIDS and Behavior, 19*(10), 1860–1874. https://doi.org/10.1007/s10461-015-1009-y

Beck, C., McSweeney, J. C., Richards, K. C., Roberson, P. K., Tsai, P.-F., & Souder, E. (2010). Challenges in tailored intervention research. *Nursing Outlook, 58*(2), 104–110. https://doi.org/10.1016/j.outlook.2009.10.004

Boudewyns, V., Paquin, R. S., Uhrig, J. D., Badal, H., August, E., & Stryker, J. E. (2018). An interrupted time series evaluation of the testing makes us stronger HIV campaign for Black gay and bisexual men in the United States. *Journal of Health Communication, 0*(0), 1–9. https://doi.org/10.1080/10810730.2018.1528318

Calabrese, S. K., Kalwicz, D. A., Dovidio, J. F., Rao, S., Modrakovic, D. X., Boone, C. A., Magnus, M., Kharfen, M., Patel, V. V., & Zea, M. C. (2023). Targeted social marketing of PrEP and the stigmatization of black sexual minority men. *PLoS One, 18*(5), e0285329. https://doi.org/10.1371/journal.pone.0285329

Centers for Disease Control and Prevention. (2018). *Preexposure prophylaxis for the prevention of HIV infection in the United States-2017 update clinical practice guideline*. https://www.cdc.gov/hiv/pdf/risk/prep/cdc-hiv-prep-guidelines-2017.pdf

Dangerfield, D. T., II. (2023). A principal investigator as a PrEP-using peer change agent for HIV prevention among Black gay and bisexual men: An autoethnography. *International Journal of Environmental Research and Public Health, 20*(7), Article 7. https://doi.org/10.3390/ijerph20075309

Dangerfield, D. T., II, & Anderson, J. N. (2024). A scripted, PrEP-using peer change agent improves perceived risk for HIV and willingness to accept referrals quickly among Black sexual minority men: Preliminary findings from POSSIBLE. *AIDS and Behavior, 28*, 2156–2165. https://doi.org/10.1007/s10461-024-04313-2

Dangerfield, D. T., II, Harawa, N. T., Smith, L. R., Jeffries, W. L., Baezconde-Garbanati, L., & Bluthenthal, R. (2018). Latent classes of sexual risk among Black men who have sex with men and women. *Archives of Sexual Behavior, 47*(7), 2071–2080. https://doi.org/10.1007/s10508-017-1142-y

Dangerfield, D. T., II, Kuo, I., Magnus, M., Beauchamp, G., Fields, S. D., Nelson, L., Shoptaw, S., Wilton, L., & Wheeler, D. P. (2021). Sexual risk profiles among Black sexual minority men: Implications for targeted PrEP messaging. *Archives of Sexual Behavior, 50*(7), 2947–2954. https://doi.org/10.1007/s10508-021-02066-w

Dangerfield, D. T., II, Anderson, J. N., Wylie, C., Arrington-Sanders, R., Bluthenthal, R. N., Beyrer, C., & Farley, J. E. (2022). Refining a multicomponent intervention to increase perceived HIV risk and PrEP initiation: Focus group study among Black sexual minority men. *JMIR Formative Research, 6*(8), e34181. https://doi.org/10.2196/34181

Dangerfield, D. T., II, Davis, G., Pandian, V., & Anderson, J. N. (2023). Using motivational interviewing to increase HIV PrEP initiation and adherence: A scoping review. *Prevention Science., 24*, 1365–1375. https://doi.org/10.1007/s11121-023-01554-w

Elion, R. A., Kabiri, M., Mayer, K. H., Wohl, D. A., Cohen, J., Beaubrun, A. C., & Altice, F. L. (2019). Estimated impact of targeted pre-exposure prophylaxis: Strategies for men who have sex with men in the United States. *International Journal of Environmental Research and Public Health, 16*(9), 1592. https://doi.org/10.3390/ijerph16091592

Ezennia, O., Geter, A., & Smith, D. K. (2019). The PrEP care continuum and Black men who have sex with men: A scoping review of published data on awareness, uptake, adherence, and retention in PrEP Care. *AIDS and Behavior, 23*(10), 2654–2673. https://doi.org/10.1007/s10461-019-02641-2

Habarta, N., Boudewyns, V., Badal, H., Johnston, J., Uhrig, J., Green, D., Ruddle, P., Rosenthal, J., & Stryker, J. E. (2017). CDC'S Testing Makes Us Stronger (TMUS) Campaign: Was campaign exposure associated with HIV testing behavior among Black gay and bisexual men? *AIDS Education and Prevention, 29*(3), 228–240.

Hoots, B. E., Finlayson, T., Nerlander, L., Paz-Bailey, G., Wortley, P., Todd, J., Sato, K., Flynn, C., German, D., Fukuda, D., Doherty, R., Wittke, C., Prachand, N., Benbow, N., Jimenez, A. D., Poe, J., Sheu, S., Novoa, A., Al-Tayyib, A., Xia, M., et al. (2016). Willingness to take, use of, and indications for pre-exposure prophylaxis among men who have sex with men—20 US cities, 2014. *Clinical Infectious Diseases, 63*(5), 672–677. https://doi.org/10.1093/cid/ciw367

Hosek, S. G. (2013). HIV pre-exposure prophylaxis diffusion and implementation issues in nonclinical settings. *American Journal of Preventive Medicine, 44*(1), S129–S132. https://doi.org/10.1016/j.amepre.2012.09.032

Hosek, S. G., Lemos, D., Hotton, A. L., Fernandez, M. I., Telander, K., Footer, D., & Bell, M. (2015). An HIV intervention tailored for Black young men who have sex with men in the House Ball Community. *AIDS Care, 27*(3), 355–362. https://doi.org/10.1080/09540121.2014.963016

Jones, K. T., Gray, P., Whiteside, Y. O., Wang, T., Bost, D., Dunbar, E., Foust, E., & Johnson, W. D. (2008). Evaluation of an HIV prevention intervention adapted for Black men who have sex with men. *American Journal of Public Health, 98*(6), 1043–1050. https://doi.org/10.2105/AJPH.2007.120337

Juusola, J. L., Brandeau, M. L., Owens, D. K., & Bendavid, E. (2012). The cost-effectiveness of preexposure prophylaxis for HIV prevention in the United States in men who have sex with men. *Annals of Internal Medicine, 156*(8), 541. https://doi.org/10.7326/0003-4819-156-8-201204170-00001

Kreuter, M. W., & Wray, R. J. (2003). Tailored and targeted health communication: Strategies for enhancing information relevance. *American Journal of Health Behavior, 27*(1), S227–S232.

Kreuter, M. W., Oswald, D. L., Bull, F. C., & Clark, E. M. (2000). Are tailored health education materials always more effective than non-tailored materials? *Health Education Research, 15*(3), 305–315. https://doi.org/10.1093/her/15.3.305

Kreuter, M. W., Lukwago, S. N., Bucholtz, D. C., Clark, E. M., & Sanders-Thompson, V. (2003). Achieving cultural appropriateness in health promotion programs: Targeted and tailored approaches. *Health Education & Behavior, 30*(2), 133–146. https://doi.org/10.1177/1090198102251021

Krueger, R. A., & Casey, M. A. (2014). *Focus groups: A practical guide for applied research*. Sage.

Lancki, N., Almirol, E., Alon, L., McNulty, M., & Schneider, J. A. (2018). Preexposure prophylaxis guidelines have low sensitivity for identifying seroconverters in a sample of young Black MSM in Chicago. *AIDS, 32*(3), 383–392. https://doi.org/10.1097/QAD.0000000000001710

Marshall, B. D. L., Goedel, W. C., King, M. R. F., Singleton, A., Durham, D. P., Chan, P. A., Townsend, J. P., & Galvani, A. P. (2018). Potential effectiveness of long-acting injectable preexposure prophylaxis for HIV prevention in men who have sex with men: A modelling study. *The Lancet. HIV, 5*(9), e498–e505. https://doi.org/10.1016/S2352-3018(18)30097-3

Miller, W. R., & Rollnick, S. (2009). Ten things that motivational interviewing is not. *Behavioural and Cognitive Psychotherapy, 37*(2), 129–140. https://doi.org/10.1017/S1352465809005128

Miller, W. R., & Rollnick, S. (2012). *Motivational interviewing: Helping people change*. Guilford Press.

Moitra, E., van den Berg, J. J., Sowemimo-Coker, G., Chau, S., Nunn, A., & Chan, P. A. (2020). Open pilot trial of a brief motivational interviewing-based HIV pre-exposure prophylaxis intervention for men who have sex with men: Preliminary effects, and evidence of feasibility and acceptability. *AIDS Care, 32*(3), 406–410. https://doi.org/10.1080/09540121.2019.1622644

Noar, S. M., Benac, C. N., & Harris, M. S. (2007). Does tailoring matter? Meta-analytic review of tailored print health behavior change interventions. *Psychological Bulletin, 133*(4), 673–693. https://doi.org/10.1037/0033-2909.133.4.673

Noar, S. M., Harrington, N. G., & Aldrich, R. S. (2009). The role of message tailoring in the development of persuasive health communication messages. *Annals of the International Communication Association, 33*(1), 73–133. https://doi.org/10.1080/23808985.2009.11679085

Psaros, C., Haberer, J. E., Katabira, E., Ronald, A., Tumwesigye, E., Campbell, J. D., Wangisi, J., Mugwanya, K., Kintu, A., Enyakoit, M., Thomas, K. K., Donnell, D., Krows, M., Kidoguchi, L., Ware, N., Baeten, J. M., Celum, C., Bangsberg, D. R., & Safren, S. A. (2014). An intervention to support HIV preexposure prophylaxis (PrEP) adherence in HIV serodiscordant couples in Uganda. *Journal of Acquired Immune Deficiency Syndromes (1999), 66*(5), 522–529. https://doi.org/10.1097/QAI.0000000000000212

Quinn, K., Dickson-Gomez, J., Zarwell, M., Pearson, B., & Lewis, M. (2018). "A gay man and a doctor are just like, a recipe for destruction": How racism and homonegativity in healthcare settings influence PrEP uptake among young Black MSM. *AIDS and Behavior*. https://doi.org/10.1007/s10461-018-2375-z

Rogers, E. M., & Adhikarya, R. (1979). Diffusion of innovations: An up-to-date review and commentary. *Annals of the International Communication Association, 3*(1), 67–81. https://doi.org/10.1080/23808985.1979.11923754

Rogers, B. G., Whiteley, L., Haubrick, K. K., Mena, L. A., & Brown, L. K. (2019). Intervention messaging about pre-exposure prophylaxis use among young, Black sexual minority men. *AIDS Patient Care and STDs, 33*(11), 473–481. https://doi.org/10.1089/apc.2019.0139

Rolle, C.-P., Rosenberg, E. S., Siegler, A. J., Sanchez, T. H., Luisi, N., Weiss, K., Cutro, S., del Rio, C., Sullivan, P. S., & Kelley, C. F. (2017). Challenges in translating PrEP interest into uptake in an observational study of young Black MSM. *JAIDS Journal of Acquired Immune Deficiency Syndromes*, Publish Ahead of Print. https://doi.org/10.1097/QAI.0000000000001497

Rollnick, S., & Miller, W. R. (1995). What is motivational interviewing? *Behavioural and Cognitive Psychotherapy, 23*(4), 325–334. https://doi.org/10.1017/S135246580001643X

Rollnick, S., Butler, C. C., Kinnersley, P., Gregory, J., & Mash, B. (2010). Motivational interviewing. *BMJ, 340*, c1900. https://doi.org/10.1136/bmj.c1900

Schleidgen, S., Klingler, C., Bertram, T., Rogowski, W. H., & Marckmann, G. (2013). What is personalized medicine: Sharpening a vague term based on a systematic literature review. *BMC Medical Ethics, 14*(1), 55. https://doi.org/10.1186/1472-6939-14-55

Schuyler, A., Alidina, Z., Dolcini, M. M., Harper, G., Fortenberry, J. D., Singh, R., Jamil, O., Pollack, L., & Catania, J. (2021). Pre-exposure prophylaxis (PrEP) dissemination: Adapting diffusion theory to examine PrEP adoption. *AIDS and Behavior, 25*(10), 3145–3158. https://doi.org/10.1007/s10461-021-03345-2

Sullivan, P. S., Rosenberg, E. S., Sanchez, T. H., Kelley, C. F., Luisi, N., Cooper, H. L., Diclemente, R. J., Wingood, G. M., Frew, P. M., Salazar, L. F., Del Rio, C., Mulligan, M. J., & Peterson, J. L. (2015). Explaining racial disparities in HIV incidence in Black and white men who have sex with men in Atlanta, GA: A prospective observational cohort study. *Annals of Epidemiology, 25*(6), 445–454. https://doi.org/10.1016/j.annepidem.2015.03.006

Testing Makes Us Stronger. (n.d.). *Testing makes us stronger*. Retrieved April 14, 2016, from //get-tested.CDC.gov/stronger/

Tutton, R. (2012). Personalizing medicine: Futures present and past. *Social Science & Medicine, 75*(10), 1721–1728. https://doi.org/10.1016/j.socscimed.2012.07.031

Wanyonyi, K. L., Themessl-Huber, M., Humphris, G., & Freeman, R. (2011). A systematic review and meta-analysis of face-to-face communication of tailored health messages: Implications for practice. *Patient Education and Counseling, 85*(3), 348–355. https://doi.org/10.1016/j.pec.2011.02.006

Wilton, L., Herbst, J. H., Coury-Doniger, P., Painter, T. M., English, G., Alvarez, M. E., Scahill, M., Roberson, M. A., Lucas, B., Johnson, W. D., & Carey, J. W. (2009). Efficacy of an HIV/STI prevention intervention for Black men who have sex with men: Findings from the Many Men, Many Voices (3MV) Project. *AIDS and Behavior, 13*(3), 532–544. https://doi.org/10.1007/s10461-009-9529-y

Wray, T. B., Luo, X., Ke, J., Pérez, A. E., Carr, D. J., & Monti, P. M. (2019). Using smartphone survey data and machine learning to identify situational and contextual risk factors for HIV risk behavior among men who have sex with men who are not on PrEP. *Prevention Science., 20*, 904–913. https://doi.org/10.1007/s11121-019-01019-z

Young, L. E., Schumm, P., Alon, L., Bouris, A., Ferreira, M., Hill, B., Khanna, A. S., Valente, T. W., & Schneider, J. A. (2017). PrEP Chicago: A randomized controlled peer change agent intervention to promote the adoption of pre-exposure prophylaxis for HIV prevention among young Black men who have sex with men. *Clinical Trials, 1740774517730012*, 44–52. https://doi.org/10.1177/1740774517730012

Chapter 8
Addressing Sexual Health Misinformation

Chapter Objectives

1. Identify the role of health literacy on misinformation and sexual health outcomes.
2. Describe how misinformation affects sexual health among Black sexual minority men (SMM).
3. Identify ways to address sexual health information in prevention science

Health Literacy and Health Status

Health literacy generally refers to the ability to access, process, and understand health information and healthcare services to make informed health decisions (Berkman et al., 2010; Malloy-Weir et al., 2016). Health literacy involves a range of skills and resources including reading, writing, communication, and critical thinking, all of which enable individuals to understand prevention and treatment recommendations, navigate the healthcare system, and make appropriate health choices for themselves (Berkman et al., 2011; Williams et al., 1998). Health literacy also allows people to effectively share personal health information with clinicians to help them devise prevention or treatment plans (Paasche-Orlow & Wolf, 2007). High health literacy is associated with better health outcomes because it empowers people to engage in prevention behaviors, adhere to treatment recommendations, and effectively manage their health (Paasche-Orlow & Wolf, 2007; Williams et al., 1998). Conversely, low health literacy can increase vulnerability to misinformation, disease, and poor health condition management (Berkman et al., 2011; Paasche-Orlow & Wolf, 2007; Williams et al., 1998). Addressing health literacy is crucial for ensuring that everyone can fully participate in their health care and essential for improving prevention and community health.

D. T. Dangerfield II, *Prevention Science & Targeted Methods for HIV/STI Research with Black Sexual Minority Men*,
https://doi.org/10.1007/978-3-031-85130-8_8

Key Factors that Affect Health Literacy

There are several key factors that affect health literacy, including the following:

- Demographic characteristics (e.g., age, education level, socioeconomic status). Demographics influence an individual's access to education and resources and therefore their ability to understand health information. A characteristic such as age can affect familiarity with digital tools, while socioeconomic status can affect the availability of educational opportunities and health services. Racial differences in health literacy can occur due to the historical and systemic inequalities that affect educational opportunities, healthcare access, and overall treatment from clinicians (Osborn et al., 2007). For example, Black individuals often face barriers rooted in structural racism that can lead to differences in the quality of education and healthcare they receive. These disparities can limit their ability to understand and act on health information effectively. Additionally, experiences of discrimination and mistreatment within the healthcare system can limit information and foster medical mistrust, further complicating efforts to engage in prevention behaviors and make informed health decisions.
- Language barriers and communication challenges. Limited proficiency in the primary language of health information can hinder comprehension and effective communication with clinicians. Complex medical jargon and ineffective communication methods can create misunderstandings and prevent individuals from fully grasping important health information. Additionally, the use of medical jargon by clinicians without proper explanation can further exacerbate confusion and preventing patients from fully understanding their health conditions and treatment options, even among those who speak English. Effective communication strategies, such as plain language, explanation of treatment recommendations, and the use of interpreters, are essential to overcoming these barriers (Dangerfield II et al., 2021).
- Cultural barriers. Cultural factors such as personal beliefs also play a crucial role in health literacy (Shahin et al., 2019). These can create an environment of medical mistrust where individuals are reluctant to seek care or adhere to medical advice. Power dynamics within the healthcare system can also make it difficult for certain groups to voice their concerns or ask questions, further diminishing their ability to engage with health information and make informed decisions about their care (Quinn et al., 2018).
- Inadequate background information. A lack of having the basic knowledge regarding a particular health issue can make it difficult for individuals to understand health information and make informed decisions, especially for innovations such as vaccines or prophylactic medications. A lack of foundational knowledge about health issues can significantly hinder an individual's ability to understand and act on health information. This is particularly challenging with new or complex innovations, such as vaccines or prophylactic medications, where individuals may not have the necessary context to fully grasp the benefits and risks. Without a solid background in basic health concepts, people may

struggle to make informed decisions, leading to gaps in care and suboptimal health outcomes.

- Challenges navigating healthcare systems. Navigating the complexities of healthcare systems, including understanding how to access services, interpret insurance policies, and follow treatment protocols, is a critical aspect of health literacy. Individuals who are unfamiliar with these systems may find it overwhelming to obtain the care they need, leading to delays in treatment, missed appointments, and a general inability to effectively manage their health (Dawson-Rose et al., 2016). Simplifying these systems and providing clear, accessible guidance can help improve health literacy and ensure that individuals can successfully navigate their healthcare journeys.
- Technology access. In today's digital age, access to and use of technology is increasingly linked to health literacy. Limited access to digital devices, internet connectivity, and digital literacy skills can prevent individuals from utilizing online health resources, telehealth services and electronic health records. As healthcare continues to evolve with a greater emphasis on digital tools, ensuring equitable access to technology is essential for improving health literacy and enabling all individuals to engage fully in their health management.

Culture, Language, and Communication

Culture, language, and communication have key influence on health literacy, especially among Black SMM. Culture generally shapes people's health beliefs, health care attitudes, and prevention behaviors, all of which affect how they interpret health information (Airhihenbuwa et al., 2014; Timmins et al., 2021). Cultural stigma and discrimination can deter Black SMM from accessing accurate health information (Arnold et al., 2014; Arrington-Sanders et al., 2020; Quinn et al., 2018). Language and communication barriers can complicate their ability to understand health information and communicate effectively with clinicians (Fisher et al., 2018). Still, much of the language involved in prevention and treatment recommendations is not easily accessible or understandable to the general population and clinicians do not always "translate" health information in ways that are easy to understand (Golub & Myers, 2019). The intersection of racial and sexual minority status can exacerbate these challenges because these men may face compounded biases and unique health concerns that are not adequately addressed by mainstream health education. Effective communication is essential for ensuring that health information is accessible and comprehensible to diverse populations. Careful consideration to the words being used when disseminating health information is also crucial for health literacy and reducing misinformation among Black SMM (Dangerfield II et al., 2021, 2022a; Dangerfield II & Wylie, 2022). Health literacy can be improved by fostering a more inclusive healthcare environment that understands and respects the diversity of Black SMM, leading to cultural competency and less misinformation (Centers for Disease Control and Prevention, 2020; Dangerfield II et al., 2021).

Health Misinformation

Misinformation generally refers to incorrect or misleading information, mostly with unintentional harm (Mikati et al., 2023; Vraga & Bode, 2020). Some definitions of health misinformation involve strictly as false or inaccurate health-related information; others include misleading or incomplete information that may not necessarily be false but can still lead to harmful health behaviors (and outcomes). There is a lack of consensus regarding the features of misinformation regarding message intention, audience perceptions, and the scope of the information that is debatable among prevention scientists, clinicians, and public health professionals (Mikati et al., 2023; Vraga & Bode, 2020). The lack of consensus complicates efforts to develop standardized methods for identifying, tracking, and addressing misinformation, posing challenges to implementing effective public health interventions (Vraga & Bode, 2020). Still, health misinformation poses significant risks to community health through the spread of inaccurate, false, or misleading information that can interrupt prevention recommendations and intervention effects, impact decision making, and lead to harmful behaviors (Dangerfield II et al., 2022a; Garett & Young, 2022). It also undermines trust in prevention scientists, clinicians, and public health professionals, complicating efforts to manage health crises and promote effective interventions. The viral spread of misinformation via social media and other online platforms exacerbates these issues, making it difficult for accurate information to reach and influence the public (Grov et al., 2021; Sundstrom et al., 2021). Addressing sexual health misinformation requires coordinated efforts to improve health literacy and design rigorous approaches for monitoring and addressing false information (Sundstrom et al., 2021; Vraga & Bode, 2020).

Sexual Health Misinformation Among Black Sexual Minority Men

Over the past decade, my exposure to the attitudes, beliefs, and understandings of sexual health prevention behaviors among Black SMM has deepened my awareness of culturally specific forms of sexual health misinformation for this group. This insight has also informed my understanding of how these misconceptions affects their lives and how prevention scientists can effectively address them. Specifically, misinformation regarding sexuality, HIV/STI prevention, PrEP, and the research process remains prevalent for Black SMM, often leading to misconceptions that hinder effective health interventions. Identifying and addressing these inaccuracies is crucial for contemporary prevention science and supporting Black SMM with accurate sexual health information.

Sexuality Misinformation

One crucial, unaddressed piece of misinformation I have found among Black SMM is that some think that identifying as gay, bisexual, or same-sex attracted is bad, wrong, or shameful (Dangerfield II, 2023; Dangerfield II et al., 2017, 2020). Many of the men I have worked with (also evidenced in the literature) have believed this at some point in their lives even if they identify as gay or bisexual men because they received early childhood messages from family, churches, and media coupled with policies that permitted mistreatment towards sexual and gender minorities. Some scholars may not consider internalized homonegativity as misinformation. However, internalized homophobia should be included in discussions regarding misinformation because society's attitudes toward same-sex sexuality is changing, reflected by the legalization of same-sex marriage, increased bullying prevention policies, and the proliferation of same-sex families. The understandings of the mechanisms of internalized homonegativity require updates and further discussion because internalized homophobia increases drug use, sexual risk taking, and subsequent HIV/STIs among Black SMM in ways that misinformation facilitates (Ross et al., 2008, 2013; Turpin et al., 2021). The combined social and political messages that have evolved regarding same-sex sexuality suggest that internalized homophobia is based on outdated and increasingly inaccurate beliefs about sexual orientation. The evolution in societal attitudes indicates that negative perceptions of same-sex attraction are not only harmful but also misaligned with contemporary values and legal standards. Acknowledging and addressing this form of misinformation is crucial for the mental health and well-being of Black gay and bisexual men. Challenging internalized homonegativity can help reduce the stigma and discrimination that Black SMM face and facilitate even more accepting and supportive communities.

Drug Use Misinformation

Some Black SMM also believe that illicit drug use is safer in their social or sexual networks than among people they "do not know" (Dangerfield II et al., 2020; Ober et al., 2018). In my STOP study, which examined the motivations for **st**imulant and **op**ioid use Baltimore City (Dangerfield II et al., 2020), Black gay and bisexual men reported being open to using most any illicit drug that a friend or partner was using before or during sex. Some of them believed this because they directly observed the drug's effects on their friends before they use them themselves. Additionally, people also trust that their friend or sexual partner would not intentionally put them in a dangerous situation. However, drug tests among participants showed that fentanyl was present in the drugs among everyone who reported using opioids. Studies have shown that normalizing drug use in social networks increases drug use and overdose risk within the network (Bright & Sutherland, 2017; De et al., 2007; Latkin et al., 2004). This underscores the hidden dangers present even in trusted social networks.

The false sense of security can lead to unintentional exposure to highly potent and dangerous substances, increasing the risk of both HIV and overdose.

HIV/STI Prevention Misinformation

Some Black SMM will engage in strategic sexual positioning for HIV/STI prevention, as discussed in Chap. 1 (Mann et al., 2022; Ober et al., 2018). Specifically, some will only engage in oral sex or insertive anal sex to avoid HIV infection or a rectal STI because risk is relatively lower than practicing receptive anal intercourse. Some will not "bottom" (practice receptive anal sex) with partners they know are living with HIV. Chapter 1 examined the sexual epidemiology of Black SMM an examined the motivations and contexts of strategic positioning. Statistically, data show that practicing condomless receptive anal sex does confer greater HIV and STI risk than condomless insertive anal sex (Baggaley et al., 2018). The effectiveness of strategic positioning to prevent HIV or STIs among Black SMM is mixed, largely due to the high background prevalence in the community and sexual networks (Irvin et al., 2015). However, HIV risk is still generally high for Black SMM in light of suboptimal PrEP use and treatment adherence; STI risk is also high in the community regardless of sexual role preference (Scott-Sheldon & Chan, 2020). Strategic positioning creates complex sexual network that could facilitate HIV/STI transmission and drug resistant bacteria (Wilken et al., 2016). The interconnected nature of sexual networks means that individual prevention strategies may be less effective without a broader, community-level approach. Comprehensive strategies that include education, increased access to PrEP, and community engagement are crucial to reducing the risk and improving health outcomes.

HIV Testing Misinformation

I have also observed that some Black SMM literally think that HIV testing prevents HIV. For example, I have heard some Black gay men say, "*I know I'm safe from HIV because I got tested.*" Prevention scientists and clinicians overlook this language because technically, knowing your status is crucial to preventing HIV in several ways. First, knowing you are HIV negative confirms that you will not pose an HIV risk to partners and enables you to consider using PrEP to prevent disease. Second, having an HIV test confirm that you are living with HIV allows you to access necessary treatment to reduce transmission risk and improve quality of life. HIV testing to learn one's status is a key first step in the HIV continuum of prevention and care (Centers for Disease Control and Prevention, 2015). However, some men do not think about this in this way and instead have literally interpreted prevention messaging of HIV testing being akin to condom use as prevention and not adding the context of it testing as part of the prevention and care continuum. This misconception highlights the need for clearer communication about the role of HIV testing in the broader strategy of HIV prevention and care. This highlights an important but understudied area; more research is needed to understand the origins of these misconceptions and design interventions that effectively clarify the role of HIV testing within the broader continuum of prevention and care.

PrEP Misinformation

"I don't need PrEP because I'm not out here like that". Some Black gay and bisexual men believe that PrEP is only useful for those who are "highly sexually active" or "risky," whatever they assume that means, and do not consider it worth the perceived barriers to obtain and use it (Dangerfield II, 2023; Dangerfield II et al., 2022b). Attitudes towards which may be influenced by clinical guidelines targeting those with histories of condomless sex, stimulant drug use, or concurrent partners within specific time frames (Centers for Disease Control and Prevention, 2018). These guidelines are designed to help clinicians identify the best candidates for PrEP by assessing risk factors such as having a history of STIs, drug use, and not being in a monogamous relationship. This approach can inadvertently reinforce the misconception that PrEP is only for those who engage in high-risk sexual behavior rather than as a preventive medicine for anyone at potential risk of HIV. Therefore, it is crucial to communicate that PrEP can benefit a wider range of individuals beyond those traditionally considered at high risk (Dangerfield II et al., 2022a).

Understanding and addressing misinformation about the side effects of PrEP is also crucial for improving its acceptance and usage among Black SMM. Common misconceptions include exaggerated fears of severe health consequences, such as kidney damage or bone density loss, (Dangerfield II et al., 2022a; Tetteh et al., 2017) which are actually rare and generally reversible with proper medical supervision (Fonner et al., 2016). In reality, PrEP is well-tolerated by most individuals, with mild side effects like nausea or headache typically subsiding within the first few weeks of use (Fang et al., 2019). These misconceptions may stem from a lack of comprehensive education on PrEP, as well as historical distrust in the healthcare system. Misinformation about the side effects of PrEP can significantly hinder its uptake among those who could benefit from it, including Black gay men. Clear, accurate information about the safety and efficacy of PrEP, along with consistent support from clinicians, is essential to dispel myths and encourage more people to consider this effective HIV prevention method. Still, Black gay men are not necessarily wrong for being skeptical about the side effects of HIV prevention medication. Historically, the Black community has experienced prejudice and medical mistreatment, which contribute to understandable caution regarding new treatments. Additionally, concerns about potential side effects and the long-term impact of medication are valid and should be acknowledged and addressed by clinicians. Transparent communication about the benefits and risks of HIV prevention medication, along with culturally competent care, is essential to building trust and encouraging informed decision-making (Dangerfield II et al., 2022a, 2022b).

Low Perceived Risks for HIV and STIs

Some Black gay men assess their HIV/STI relative to their past or their peers that they may think have "higher" risk than they do. For example, some think that they have lower HIV vulnerability because they have relatively fewer partners than they did at earlier ages, or they compare their behaviors to their behaviors to their friends who they believe have more sex than they do and have remained HIV-negative (Dangerfield II et al., 2022b; Ober et al., 2018). These assumptions contribute to a low perception of HIV risk, which is particularly concerning given that 2017 modeling data estimated that 1 in 2 Black SMM will acquire HIV in their lifetime (Hess et al., 2017). Chapter 2 discussed the social, psychological, and epidemiological conundrum faced by Black SMM and the differences between the concepts of "risk" versus "vulnerability" for HIV/STIs. This form of misinformation persists throughout the community and contribute to the low uptake and adherence of prevention regimens. Since anyone who is having condomless sex is vulnerable, prevention scientists should emphasize that the number of partners or comparison to peers does not eliminate risk. We must also clarify who in the community are the most vulnerable to HIV. Moreover, we must also ensure that partners of people living with obtain clear messaging about their vulnerability. Efforts should focus on comprehensive education and accessible prevention strategies to address these misconceptions and reduce the incidence of HIV.

Research Misinformation

Given the extensive amount of primary data that I have collected first-hand, I have been privy to some misperceptions regarding the purpose and utility of research, particularly clinical trials methodology, among Black SMM. For example, some believe that randomization in clinical trials not "fair", despite the statistical and ethical justification we use to design and test interventions (Dangerfield II & Wylie, 2022). They believe that in interventions in which one group gets something more or different from the control group, low-resourced individuals are cheated from a beneficial opportunity that could exacerbate inequities. Theoretically driven interventions are hypothesized to provide better outcomes than control conditions (Cook & Sheets, 2011). However, despite informed consent documents, participants might be misinformed that clinical trials are social service provisions that could be expected from governmental programs and not just federally sponsored experimental studies. Chapter 9 will discuss research ethics in greater detail. Still, this is of crucial importance to address as misinformation because such beliefs can undermine trust in research and hinder participation from communities that could significantly benefit from these studies (Dangerfield II & Wylie, 2022). Educating participants about the scientific and ethical principles underlying clinical trials can help demystify the process, promote equity, and ensure that interventions are developed and tested in ways that ultimately serve the needs of Black SMM and other marginalized groups.

The Misinformation of U=U

In 2017, the Prevention Access Campaign launched the "U=U" (Undetectable = Untransmittable) campaign, endorsed by the World Health Organization, to reduce HIV stigma by emphasizing that individuals with an undetectable viral load cannot transmit the virus to their partners (Eisinger et al., 2019; National Institute of Allergy and Infectious Diseases, 2019). U=U signifies that people with HIV who achieve and maintain an undetectable viral load through consistent antiretroviral therapy cannot sexually transmit the virus to others. The campaign aims to decrease stigma among people living with HIV by educating communities about the extensive scientific evidence supporting this announcement. Despite the proliferation of its message, key information is still missing and inconsistent, which may comprise goals to decrease stigma and end the HIV epidemic. For example, sometimes practitioners say that viral suppression "nearly eliminates" HIV transmission risk, and other times the messages is that HIV "cannot be transmitted." The subtle language difference may seem inconsequential, but the difference between "low chance" and "no chance" of HIV acquisition can be very big for individuals who do not want to acquire HIV. Therefore, the message may be unappreciated if individuals perceive that HIV can be transmitted given the history of disease severity for those newly infected. Additionally, U=U might inadvertently stigmatize those who have not yet achieved an undetectable viral load given the fact that receiving an HIV diagnosis can be traumatizing for some (especially among minority communities and individuals with intersectional identities) who may need time and resources to properly access and adhere to their medication. Although the campaign is well-intentioned, we must be careful not to exclude individuals who have not yet achieved an undetectable HIV viral load from a stigma-reduction message.

Sources of Misinformation

Sexual health misinformation among Black SMM has stemmed and can stem from a several sources, including historical, social, and structural factors. Histories of mistreatment, discrimination, stigma, and violence especially among Black Americans has prevented Black SMM from receiving, understanding, and believing accurate health information that could help keep them healthy. Mistrust in the healthcare system fueled by historical and ongoing discrimination leads Black SMM to rely on their social networks for health information (Quinn et al., 2020). Consequently, some appraise their health risks relative to others or rely upon their social networks (or peers, Chap. 6) to learn about health. Additionally, race-based and sexuality stigma sometimes prevent open discussions about sexual health between Black gay men and their clinicians, contributing to misinformation (Quinn et al., 2018). Limited access to culturally competent clinicians can also exacerbate the spread of incorrect information. Social media, news, and internet sources can also propagate myths and inaccuracies about HIV/STIs (Grov et al., 2021; Westberry et al., 2023). Addressing these issues requires targeted health communication strategies and community engagement to ensure accurate and relevant information reaches Black gay men. Therefore, a focus on dismantling misinformation is crucial to improving the health for Black SMM.

The Role of Prevention Science in Addressing Misinformation

Prevention science plays a crucial role in addressing sexual health misinformation by designing and implementing evidence-based communication strategies that are targeted to the community. We discussed the crucial role of targeted communication in Chap. 7. Prevention scientists can conduct research to identify the sources and types of misinformation prevalent within different populations, allowing for targeted interventions that directly address and debunk specific myths and misconceptions. Another effective approach to reduce health misinformation is to improve health literacy by providing accurate, accessible, and culturally responsive information through multiple channels, including social media, community-based programs, and clinicians. We must maintain consistency regarding messaging and provide as many details as possible to decrease misinformation, stigma, and ultimately HIV. Collaborating with community leaders and trusted influencers can also amplify the reach and impact of accurate health messages. Additionally, integrating testimonials from individuals who have successfully utilized HIV prevention methods can provide relatable and persuasive narratives. It is essential to maintain consistency in messaging and provide comprehensive details to decrease misinformation, reduce stigma, and ultimately lower the incidence of HIV. By continuously engaging with the community and adapting strategies based on feedback, prevention scientists can create a more informed and health-literate public.

Of note, prevention scientists should prioritize building trust between healthcare systems and Black SMM. This can be achieved by engaging in transparent, two-way communication and involving community members in the development and dissemination of health messages. Fostering an environment of trust and collaboration can help prevention scientists effectively counteract misinformation and promote the adoption of accurate health behaviors. Continuous evaluation and adaptation of these strategies, based on feedback and emerging trends, will enhance their effectiveness in combating health misinformation over time.

Using Peers to Address Misinformation

Chapter 6 discussed the important role of peer change agents (PCAs) on health information sharing and decision-making among Black SMM. POSSIBLE involved two sessions with a PCA who used a motivational interview-based script to identify participants' goals and values, discuss sexual behaviors, and identifies HIV and PrEP misinformation (Dangerfield II et al., 2024). The intervention utilizes a mobile app called "PrEPme®" to encourage users to record their sexual risk behaviors and work with a PCA in a motivational interview-based conversation to review the diary and assess their interest in PrEP. The PrEP-using PCA intentionally targeted opportunities to dispel misinformation as a professional and as a patient to for those who were ambivalent towards PrEP. The key focus here was the scripts that identify sources of misinformation and the language that circumvents misinformation between the participants and the peer that subsequently encourages individuals to accept a PrEP referral. Peers (or peer change agents) can play a pivotal role in addressing sexual health misinformation among Black gay men by leveraging their shared experiences and cultural understanding to foster trust and credibility. Moreover, peers can serve as role models and demonstrate health behaviors and ways to navigate challenges associated with adhering to prevention recommendations. Given their shared identities, experiences, and challenges, peers can facilitate and process open discussions about sexual health in non-stigmatizing ways for Black SMM (Dangerfield II, 2023; Kelly, 2004; Quinn et al., 2020). They can provide accurate and culturally relevant information, dispelling myths and misconceptions about HIV/STIs and other sexual health issues, as well as disclose personal experiences that disarm Black SMM from anticipated stigma or discrimination from healthcare providers (Dangerfield II et al., 2018, 2022a, 2022b). These interactions can be particularly effective in promoting the use of preventive measures such as PrEP, regular testing, and treatment adherence. Peers (or PCAs) can enhance the reach and impact of sexual health programs by bridging the gap between clinicians and the community.

Conclusion

Unique historical, social, and cultural challenges in accessing and understanding health information affects health literacy and misinformation among Black SMM. The proliferation of misinformation exacerbates these issues by spreading false or misleading health information especially on social media. Health literacy programs should help Black SMM critically evaluate online information and respond to the information requests of sexual and racial minorities in health communication strategies. Culturally responsive health education programs, increased representation of minority groups in prevention science, and community-based interventions can build trust and reduce misinformation for this community. These measures aim to empower racial and sexual minority men with the knowledge and resources needed to make informed health decisions.

Raised Questions

1. What are the most effective words needed to improve sexual health literacy and communicate disease vulnerability among Black SMM?
2. What are more ways that trust and reduce misinformation risk can be built between prevention scientists, clinicians, and the community?
3. How can technology, including social media and artificial intelligence, be used to address misinformation?

Chapter Summary

This chapter focused on the crucial role of health literacy in combating sexual health misinformation, particularly among Black SMM. The chapter described how low health literacy can lead to misinformation and increased vulnerability to diseases like HIV and STIs. Key factors impacting health literacy include demographic characteristics, language and communication barriers, and limited access to technology. The chapter emphasized that misinformation is a significant barrier to effective sexual health interventions, often exacerbated by social media and mistrust in the healthcare system (and social services). Addressing sexual health misinformation among Black SMM requires a multi-faceted approach, including improving health literacy through culturally responsive education, enhancing communication strategies, and leveraging community-based interventions. This chapter also discussed the importance of using peers as change agents to dispel myths and promote accurate health information within the community. The chapter called for increased efforts to build trust between healthcare providers and marginalized communities to reduce misinformation and improve health outcomes for Black SMM.

Key Points

1. **Health literacy**: The ability of individuals to access, process, and understand health information in order to make informed health decisions. Health literacy encompasses skills such as reading, writing, communication, and critical thinking. Factors such as age, socioeconomic status, and education level significantly affect an individual's ability to understand and use health information, ultimately influencing health outcomes.

2. **Language, culture, and communication barriers**: Cultural factors such as personal beliefs and power dynamics, influence health literacy and can create mistrust in the healthcare system, particularly among Black SMM. Challenges understanding complex medical jargon can also prevent effective communication between patients and clinicians, leading to misunderstandings and misinformation.
3. **Misinformation**: Incorrect or misleading information that can negatively affect health behaviors and outcomes. In the context of sexual health, misinformation can lead to harmful behaviors and hinder the effectiveness of public health interventions.
4. **The role of peers on health literacy and misinformation**: Peers can serve as credible sources of information and help bridge gaps between the healthcare system and marginalized populations.
5. **Culturally responsive health communication**: Health communication strategies that are tailored to the cultural, social, and linguistic needs of Black SMM are still needed to effectively convey health information and reduce misinformation. Building trust between clinicians and Black SMM is essential to help combat misinformation and improve health outcomes.

References

Airhihenbuwa, C. O., Ford, C. L., & Iwelunmor, J. I. (2014). Why culture matters in health interventions: Lessons from HIV/AIDS stigma and NCDs. *Health Education & Behavior, 41*(1), 78–84. https://doi.org/10.1177/1090198113487199

Arnold, E. A., Rebchook, G. M., & Kegeles, S. M. (2014). "Triply cursed": Racism, homophobia, and HIV-related stigma are barriers to regular HIV testing, treatment adherence, and disclosure among young Black gay men. *Culture, Health & Sexuality, 16*(6), 710–722. https://doi.org/10.1080/13691058.2014.905706

Arrington-Sanders, R., Hailey-Fair, K., Wirtz, A. L., Morgan, A., Brooks, D., Castillo, M., Trexler, C., Kwait, J., Dowshen, N., Galai, N., Beyrer, C., & Celentano, D. (2020). Role of structural marginalization, HIV stigma, and mistrust on HIV prevention and treatment among young Black Latinx men who have sex with men and transgender women: Perspectives from youth Service Providers. *AIDS Patient Care and STDs, 34*(1), 7–15. https://doi.org/10.1089/apc.2019.0165

Baggaley, R. F., Owen, B. N., Silhol, R., Anton, P., McGowan, I., van der Straten, A., Dang, Q., Swann, E. M., Shacklett, B., & Boily, M.-C. (2018, October). *Per Act HIV transmission risk through anal intercourse: An updated systematic review and meta-analysis*. HIV Research for Prevention, Mardi. http://www.natap.org/2018/HIVR4P/BaggaleyEtAlPosterR4P_2018.pdf

Berkman, N. D., Davis, T. C., & McCormack, L. (2010). Health literacy: What is it? *Journal of Health Communication, 15*(sup2), 9–19. https://doi.org/10.1080/10810730.2010.499985

Berkman, N. D., Sheridan, S. L., Donahue, K. E., Halpern, D. J., & Crotty, K. (2011). Low health literacy and health outcomes: An updated systematic review. *Annals of Internal Medicine, 155*(2), 97–107. https://doi.org/10.7326/0003-4819-155-2-201107190-00005

Bright, D. A., & Sutherland, R. (2017). "Just doing a favor for a friend": The social supply of ecstasy through friendship networks. *Journal of Drug Issues, 47*(3), 492–504. https://doi.org/10.1177/0022042617704004

Centers for Disease Control and Prevention. (2015). *HIV testing | HIV/AIDS | CDC*. http://www.cdc.gov/hiv/testing/index.html

Centers for Disease Control and Prevention. (2018). *Preexposure prophylaxis for the prevention of HIV infection in the United States-2017 Update Clinical Practice Guideline*. https://www.cdc.gov/hiv/pdf/risk/prep/cdc-hiv-prep-guidelines-2017.pdf

Centers for Disease Control and Prevention. (2020, April 6). *Taking a Sexual History | For Health Care Providers | Transforming Health | Clinicians | HIV | CDC*. https://www.cdc.gov/hiv/clinicians/transforming-health/health-care-providers/sexual-history.html

Cook, C., & Sheets, C. (2011). Clinical equipoise and personal equipoise: Two necessary ingredients for reducing bias in manual therapy trials. *The Journal of Manual & Manipulative Therapy, 19*(1), 55–57. https://doi.org/10.1179/106698111X12899036752014

Dangerfield, D. T., II. (2023). A principal investigator as a PrEP-using peer change agent for HIV prevention among Black gay and bisexual men: An autoethnography. *International Journal of Environmental Research and Public Health, 20*(7), 5309. https://doi.org/10.3390/ijerph20075309

Dangerfield, D. T., II, & Wylie, C. (2022). Identifying ethical and culturally responsive research activities to build trust and improve participation of Black sexual minority men in pre-exposure prophylaxis telehealth clinical trials: Qualitative Study. *JMIR Human Factors, 9*(1), e28798. https://doi.org/10.2196/28798

Dangerfield, D. T., II, Smith, L. R., Anderson, J. N., Bruce, O. J., Farley, J., & Bluthenthal, R. (2017). Sexual positioning practices and sexual risk among Black gay and bisexual men: A life course perspective. *AIDS and Behavior, 22*(6), 1919–1931. https://doi.org/10.1007/s10461-017-1948-6

Dangerfield, D. T., II, Harawa, N. T., McWells, C., Hilliard, C., & Bluthenthal, R. N. (2018). Exploring the preferences of a culturally congruent, peer-based HIV prevention intervention for Black men who have sex with men. *Sexual Health, 15*(5), 424–430. https://doi.org/10.1071/SH18057

Dangerfield, D. T., II, Heidari, O., Cooper, J., Allen, S., & Lucas, G. M. (2020). Motivations for opioid and stimulant use among drug using black sexual minority men: A life course perspective. *Drug and Alcohol Dependence, 215*, 108224. https://doi.org/10.1016/j.drugalcdep.2020.108224

Dangerfield, D. T., II, Cooper, J., Heidari, O., Allen, S., Winder, T. J. A., & Lucas, G. M. (2021). Nursing and health care preferences among opioid and stimulant using Black sexual minority men: An exploratory study. *Journal of the Association of Nurses in AIDS Care, 32*(5), e30–e39. https://doi.org/10.1097/JNC.0000000000000201

Dangerfield, D. T., II, Lipson, A., & Anderson, J. N. (2022a). HIV PrEP clinician communication preferences among Black sexual minority men. *AIDS Education and Prevention, 34*(2), 168–181. https://doi.org/10.1521/aeap.2022.34.2.168

Dangerfield, D. T., II, Anderson, J. N., Wylie, C., Arrington-Sanders, R., Bluthenthal, R. N., Beyrer, C., & Farley, J. E. (2022b). Refining a multicomponent intervention to increase perceived HIV risk and PrEP initiation: Focus group study among Black sexual minority men. *JMIR Formative Research, 6*(8), e34181. https://doi.org/10.2196/34181

Dangerfield, D. T., II, Anderson, J. N., Wylie, C., Bluthenthal, R., Beyrer, C., & Farley, J. E. (2024). A multicomponent intervention (POSSIBLE) to improve perceived risk for HIV among Black sexual minority men: Feasibility and preliminary effectiveness pilot study. *JMIR Human Factors, 11*(1), e54739. https://doi.org/10.2196/54739

Dawson-Rose, C., Cuca, Y. P., Webel, A. R., Solís Báez, S. S., Holzemer, W. L., Rivero-Méndez, M., Sanzero Eller, L., Reid, P., Johnson, M. O., Kemppainen, J., Reyes, D., Nokes, K., Nicholas, P. K., Matshediso, E., Mogobe, K. D., Sabone, M. B., Ntsayagae, E. I., Shaibu, S., Corless, I. B., Lindgren, T., et al. (2016). Building trust and relationships between patients and providers: An essential complement to health literacy in HIV care. *Journal of the Association of Nurses in AIDS Care, 27*(5), 574–584. https://doi.org/10.1016/j.jana.2016.03.001

De, P., Cox, J., Boivin, J.-F., Platt, R. W., & Jolly, A. M. (2007). The importance of social networks in their association to drug equipment sharing among injection drug users: A review. *Addiction, 102*(11), 1730–1739. https://doi.org/10.1111/j.1360-0443.2007.01936.x

Eisinger, R. W., Dieffenbach, C. W., & Fauci, A. S. (2019). HIV viral load and transmissibility of HIV infection: Undetectable equals untransmittable. *JAMA, 321*(5), 451–452. https://doi.org/10.1001/jama.2018.21167

Fang, W., Mphoyi, B. I., Motake, D. R., Liu, J., Li, W., Mei, F., Lai, S., & Wang, J. (2019). Efficacy, adherence and side effects of PrEP for HIV-1 prevention. *International Journal of Biology, 11*(4), 80. https://doi.org/10.5539/ijb.v11n4p80

Fisher, C. B., Fried, A. L., Macapagal, K., & Mustanski, B. (2018). Patient–provider communication barriers and facilitators to HIV and STI preventive services for adolescent MSM. *AIDS and Behavior, 22*(10), 3417–3428. https://doi.org/10.1007/s10461-018-2081-x

Fonner, V. A., Dalglish, S. L., Kennedy, C. E., Baggaley, R., O'Reilly, K. R., Koechlin, F. M., Rodolph, M., Hodges-Mameletzis, I., & Grant, R. M. (2016). Effectiveness and safety of oral HIV preexposure prophylaxis for all populations. *AIDS (London, England), 30*(12), 1973–1983. https://doi.org/10.1097/QAD.0000000000001145

Garett, R., & Young, S. D. (2022). The impact of misinformation and health literacy on HIV prevention and service usage. *Journal of the Association of Nurses in AIDS Care, 33*(1), e1. https://doi.org/10.1097/JNC.0000000000000298

Golub, S. A., & Myers, J. E. (2019). Next-wave HIV pre-exposure prophylaxis implementation for gay and bisexual men. *AIDS Patient Care and STDs, 33*(6), 253–261. https://doi.org/10.1089/apc.2018.0290

Grov, C., Westmoreland, D. A., D'Angelo, A. B., Johnson, J., Nash, D., Daskalakis, D. C., & the Together 5000 team. (2021). Marketing of tenofovir disoproxil fumarate (TDF) lawsuits and social media misinformation campaigns' impact on PrEP uptake among gender and sexual minority individuals. *AIDS and Behavior, 25*(5), 1396–1404. https://doi.org/10.1007/s10461-020-02977-0

Hess, K. L., Hu, X., Lansky, A., Mermin, J., & Hall, H. I. (2017). Lifetime risk of a diagnosis of HIV infection in the United States. *Annals of Epidemiology, 27*(4), 238–243. https://doi.org/10.1016/j.annepidem.2017.02.003

Irvin, R., Vallabhaneni, S., Scott, H., Williams, J. K., Wilton, L., Li, X., Buchbinder, S., & 061, on behalf of H. (2015). Examining levels of risk behaviors among Black men who have sex with men (MSM) and the association with HIV acquisition. *PLoS One, 10*(2), e0118281. https://doi.org/10.1371/journal.pone.0118281

Kelly, J. A. (2004). Popular opinion leaders and HIV prevention peer education: Resolving discrepant findings, and implications for the development of effective community programmes. *AIDS Care, 16*(2), 139–150. https://doi.org/10.1080/09540120410001640986

Latkin, C. A., Hua, W., & Tobin, K. (2004). Social network correlates of self-reported nonfatal overdose. *Drug and Alcohol Dependence, 73*(1), 61–67. https://doi.org/10.1016/j.drugalcdep.2003.09.005

Malloy-Weir, L. J., Charles, C., Gafni, A., & Entwistle, V. (2016). A review of health literacy: Definitions, interpretations, and implications for policy initiatives. *Journal of Public Health Policy, 37*(3), 334–352. https://doi.org/10.1057/jphp.2016.18

Mann, L. M., Kelley, C. F., Siegler, A. J., Stephenson, R., & Sullivan, P. S. (2022). Seroadaptive strategy patterns of young Black gay, bisexual, and other men who have sex with men in Atlanta, Georgia. *JAIDS Journal of Acquired Immune Deficiency Syndromes, 89*(1), 40–48. https://doi.org/10.1097/QAI.0000000000002816

Mikati, I. K. E., Hoteit, R., Harb, T., Zein, O. E., Piggott, T., Melki, J., Mustafa, R. A., & Akl, E. A. (2023). Defining misinformation and related terms in health-related literature: Scoping review. *Journal of Medical Internet Research, 25*(1), e45731. https://doi.org/10.2196/45731

National Institute of Allergy and Infectious Diseases. (2019, May 21). *HIV Undetectable=Untransmittable (U=U), or Treatment as Prevention*. https://www.niaid.nih.gov/diseases-conditions/treatment-prevention

Ober, A. J., Dangerfield, D. T., II, Shoptaw, S., Ryan, G., Stucky, B., & Friedman, S. R. (2018). Using a "Positive Deviance" framework to discover adaptive risk reduction behaviors among high-risk HIV negative Black men who have sex with men. *AIDS and Behavior, 22*(5), 1699–1712. https://doi.org/10.1007/s10461-017-1790-x

Osborn, C. Y., Paasche-Orlow, M. K., Davis, T. C., & Wolf, M. S. (2007). Health literacy: An overlooked factor in understanding HIV health disparities. *American Journal of Preventive Medicine, 33*(5), 374–378. https://doi.org/10.1016/j.amepre.2007.07.022

Paasche-Orlow, M. K., & Wolf, M. S. (2007). The causal pathways linking health literacy to health outcomes. *American Journal of Health Behavior, 31*(1), S19–S26.

Quinn, K., Dickson-Gomez, J., Zarwell, M., Pearson, B., & Lewis, M. (2018). "A gay man and a doctor are just like, a recipe for destruction": How racism and homonegativity in healthcare settings influence PrEP uptake among young Black MSM. *AIDS and Behavior, 23*, 1951–1963. https://doi.org/10.1007/s10461-018-2375-z

Quinn, K. G., Christenson, E., Spector, A., Amirkhanian, Y., & Kelly, J. A. (2020). The influence of peers on PrEP perceptions and use among young Black gay, bisexual, and other men who have sex with men: A qualitative examination. *Archives of Sexual Behavior., 49*, 2129–2143. https://doi.org/10.1007/s10508-019-01593-x

Ross, M. W., Rosser, B. R. S., Neumaier, E. R., & Team, the P. C. (2008). The relationship of internalized homonegativity to unsafe sexual behavior in HIV seropositive men who have sex with men. *AIDS Education and Prevention: Official Publication of the International Society for AIDS Education, 20*(6), 547–557. https://doi.org/10.1521/aeap.2008.20.6.547

Ross, M. W., Kajubi, P., Mandel, J. S., McFarland, W., & Raymond, H. F. (2013). Internalized homonegativity/homophobia is associated with HIV-risk behaviours among Ugandan gay and bisexual men. *International Journal of STD & AIDS, 24*(5), 409–413. https://doi.org/10.1177/0956462412472793

Scott-Sheldon, L. A. J., & Chan, P. A. (2020). Increasing sexually transmitted infections in the U.S.: A call for action for research, clinical, and public health practice. *Archives of Sexual Behavior, 49*(1), 13–17. https://doi.org/10.1007/s10508-019-01584-y

Shahin, W., Kennedy, G. A., & Stupans, I. (2019). The impact of personal and cultural beliefs on medication adherence of patients with chronic illnesses: A systematic review. *Patient Preference and Adherence, 13*, 1019–1035. https://doi.org/10.2147/PPA.S212046

Sundstrom, B., Cartmell, K. B., White, A. A., Well, H., Pierce, J. Y., & Brandt, H. M. (2021). Correcting HPV vaccination misinformation online: Evaluating the HPV vaccination *NOW* social media campaign. *Vaccine, 9*(4), 352. https://doi.org/10.3390/vaccines9040352

Tetteh, R. A., Yankey, B. A., Nartey, E. T., Lartey, M., Leufkens, H. G. M., & Dodoo, A. N. O. (2017). Pre-exposure prophylaxis for HIV prevention: Safety concerns. *Drug Safety, 40*(4), 273–283. https://doi.org/10.1007/s40264-017-0505-6

Timmins, L., Schneider, J. A., Chen, Y.-T., Goedel, W. C., Brewer, R., Callander, D., Knox, J., Eavou, R., Hanson, H., & Duncan, D. T. (2021). Sexual identity, sexual behavior and pre-exposure prophylaxis in Black cisgender sexual minority men: The N2 Cohort Study in Chicago. *AIDS and Behavior., 25*, 3327–3336. https://doi.org/10.1007/s10461-021-03246-4

Turpin, R., Dyer, T., Watson, L., & Mayer, K. (2021). Classes of sexual identity, homophobia, and sexual risk among Black sexual minorities in HPTN 061. *The Journal of Sex Research, 58*(5), 638–647. https://doi.org/10.1080/00224499.2021.1886228

Vraga, E. K., & Bode, L. (2020). Defining misinformation and understanding its bounded nature: Using expertise and evidence for describing misinformation. *Political Communication, 37*(1), 136–144. https://doi.org/10.1080/10584609.2020.1716500

Westberry, C., Palmer, X.-L., & Potter, L. (2023). Social media and health misinformation: A literature review. In K. Arai (Ed.), *Proceedings of the Future Technologies Conference (FTC) 2023,3*, 404–418. Springer Nature Switzerland. https://doi.org/10.1007/978-3-031-47457-6_26

Wilken, J. A., Ried, C., Rickett, P., Arno, J. N., Mendez, Y., Harrison, R. J., Wohlfeiler, D., Bauer, H. M., Joyce, M. P., Switzer, W. M., Heneine, W., Shankar, A., & Mark, K. E. (2016). Occupational HIV transmission among male adult film performers—multiple states, 2014. *MMWR. Morbidity and Mortality Weekly Report, 65*(5), 110–114. https://doi.org/10.15585/mmwr.mm6505a3

Williams, M. V., Baker, D. W., Parker, R. M., & Nurss, J. R. (1998). Relationship of functional health literacy to patients' knowledge of their chronic disease: A study of patients with hypertension and diabetes. *Archives of Internal Medicine, 158*(2), 166–172. https://doi.org/10.1001/archinte.158.2.166

Chapter 9
Ethical Research Conduct with Black Sexual Minority Men

Chapter Objectives

1. Highlight the general importance of ethical research conduct in prevention science.
2. Describe contemporary ethical issues in prevention science conduct with Black sexual minority men (SMM).
3. Identify strategies to maximize ethical conduct with racial and sexual minority men.

The Importance of Ethical Research Conduct in Prevention Science

Research ethics involve principles and standards that guide scientists to conduct studies in responsible ways so that participants are safe and protected, that the research process has integrity, and that the science is credible (Israel & Hay, 2006). The Belmont Report outlines fundamental ethical principles such as respect for persons, beneficence, and justice, which are the foundation of ethical guidelines for human subjects research (National Commission for the Protection of Human Subjects of Biomedical and Behavioral Research, 1979). Respect for persons requires that researchers obtain informed consent from participants, protect their autonomy, and ensure their confidentiality. Beneficence mandates that researchers maximize the benefits and minimize potential harms of the research, conduct thorough risk assessments, and implement necessary protections against those risks. Justice ensures equitable selection of research participants and avoiding exploiting vulnerable populations (Fisher, 2016; National Commission for the Protection of

D. T. Dangerfield II, *Prevention Science & Targeted Methods for HIV/STI Research with Black Sexual Minority Men*,
https://doi.org/10.1007/978-3-031-85130-8_9

Human Subjects of Biomedical and Behavioral Research, 1979). Ethical research conduct is key to ensuring that the prevention science adheres to the highest standards of integrity, methodology, and responsibility and maximizes benefits to society (World Health Organization, 2017).

Moreover, ethical research conduct requires methodological transparency to verify results and improve replication (Moravcsik, 2019; World Health Organization, 2017). In addition to these principles, ethical prevention science includes a commitment to the welfare of the communities involved in or affected by the research (World Health Organization, 2017). Adhering to ethical standards also helps improve and maintain trust from the public and fosters the design of safe, effective, reliable, and equitable prevention interventions (Fisher, 2016). Therefore, it is important to consider the potential social, cultural, and economic impacts of the research and minimize any negative consequences.

Focus on Ethical Conduct with Black Sexual Minority Men

Focus on ethical research conduct with Black sexual minority men (SMM) is crucial given their histories and present day experiences of marginalization, discrimination, and violence in society. Personal experiences of discrimination, stigma, and violence also affect trust in prevention science and medicine (Arnold et al., 2014; Arrington-Sanders et al., 2020; Cahill et al., 2017). Background medical and research mistrust is salient among Black SMM given these narratives, other atrocities, and unethical practices of the medical/research system in studies including (but not limited to) the well-known Tuskegee Syphilis Study (Dangerfield II & Wylie, 2022; Scharff et al., 2010). These experiences increase research mistrust and apprehension to participate in prevention and treatment behaviors as well as research (Dangerfield II et al., 2024a; Dangerfield II & Wylie, 2022). It also decreases willingness for Black SMM to disclose personal or sensitive information to researchers in studies, especially to those who are not culturally similar (Dangerfield II et al., 2022b, 2021a). Therefore, ethical conduct with Black SMM involves an intentional focus to ensure that their informed consent, privacy, and safety are guaranteed. Ethical research practices ensure that the findings are not only scientifically sound but also socially responsible and promote health equity and justice. Ethical research conduct helps ensure that the experiences and needs of the community are accurately represented (World Health Organization, 2017), which is imperative to produce valid and reliable data that can inform public health policies and interventions for the community. This, in turn, can lead to more effective and targeted health initiatives (as discussed in Chap. 7), addressing sexual health issues and other health disparities. Moreover, recommendations from ethical prevention science may be more accepted by Black SMM than studies done haphazardly or for general populations (Dangerfield II et al., 2022b; Dangerfield II et al., 2021b; Dangerfield II & Wylie, 2022).

Ethical Issues in Sexual Health Prevention Science with Black Sexual Minority Men

Although ethical guidelines are established for prevention science, my targeted studies suggest that ethical guidelines should also acknowledge and addresses nuanced factors involved in research with this community (Dangerfield II et al., 2022a; Dangerfield II & Wylie, 2022). For example, traditional ethical standards may not fully consider how historical and systemic inequalities influence research participation and trust of individuals who are part of racial and sexual minority groups because these guidelines often overlook the deep-seated mistrust stemming from past abuses and discrimination in medical research for this specific group. For example, ethical guidelines for research among Black SMM are limited because there is a lack of targeted (and tailored) ethical frameworks that address the unique social, cultural, and emotional vulnerabilities of the community such as the impact of racial trauma, stigma, and discrimination on their willingness to engage in research. These guidelines often fail to address how these factors can influence consent processes, data sharing, and confidentiality concerns. There is also a need for ethical frameworks that emphasize building trust and fostering long-term relationships between researchers and Black SMM, rather than just focusing on compliance with standard procedures. Tailoring ethical considerations to reflect the lived experiences of Black SMM can help ensure that research is conducted in a way that respects their dignity, protects their rights, and promotes meaningful participation. More culturally responsive approaches that ensure prevention science approaches are respectful and meaningful regarding several issues, including using persuasive communication tactics for public health promotion, using in-group members as interventionists, and culturally responsive informed consent details. Guidelines regarding crucial research activities such as informed consent, confidentiality, and beneficence might not be specific enough to satisfy ethical conduct considerations among Black SMM and may potentially compromise the efficacy and ethical soundness of the research. Addressing these issues requires ongoing dialogue and adaptation of ethical guidelines to better protect and empower Black SMM in prevention science contexts. This chapter emphasizes the need to revisit and revise current ethical guidelines to ensure they are not only inclusive but also responsive to the unique challenges faced by Black SMM and advocates for more nuanced ethical frameworks that recognize historical and systemic barriers, incorporate culturally sensitive approaches, and prioritize trust-building in research.

Using Persuasive Communication Tactics to Encourage Health Behaviors

Chapter 2 described the crucial role of using theoretically driven approaches in prevention science to improve health behavior and public health, especially among racial and sexual minority men. However, using behavior change and learning models can raise ethical questions regarding the role of "choice" in health behavior (Rossi & Yudell, 2012), especially among a population with histories of marginalization. For example, health communication strategies guided by theoretical frameworks such as the Health Belief Model (Rosenstock, 1974) or the Extended Parallel Process Model (Witte, 1992) could be considered manipulative because they use sophisticated strategies that are intentionally designed to influence people's behaviors and decisions using fear appeals (Jacobs, 2020; Rossi & Yudell, 2012). This manipulation can occur through direct or indirect methods that subtly guides people toward specific health behaviors that align with public health priorities and not necessarily the priorities of the individual or community. Although the ultimate goal is to improve community and public health outcomes, these kinds of approaches can raise ethical concerns about the extent to which individuals' autonomy and freedom of choice are respected (Jacobs, 2020; Rossi & Yudell, 2012). Prevention campaigns can shape perceptions, attitudes, and behaviors using psychological and behavioral theories in ways that might not always be transparent to the target population. Health campaign guided by behavior change and learning models, while effective, could blur the line between informed persuasion and coercive manipulation, leading to debates about the appropriateness and morality of these interventions for minority health promotion. Moreover, persuading individuals and communities to engage in public health priority behavior is often a "top-down" approach rather than a collaborative process that prioritizes the interests and preferences of the community.

To address these concerns, ethical considerations regarding using persuasion in health promotion campaigns must involve a careful analysis of the methods and motivations to influence behavior and their potential impact on individual freedom of choice. Ethical persuasion in health promotion requires a balance between achieving public health goals and upholding individual rights and dignity (Parrott, 2008). The World Health Organization emphasizes that campaigns should be grounded in principles of respect, equity, and transparency (World Health Organization, 2017). In alignment with ethical principles, persuasive strategies must respect autonomy and ensure that individuals can make voluntary and informed decisions without deception. This means providing clear, accurate, and balanced information about the health issue, the proposed intervention(s), and their benefits and risks to the satisfaction of Black SMM (Dangerfield II et al., 2021b; Dangerfield II & Wylie, 2022). Ethical health promotion should also address power imbalances between scientists, healthcare, and the community so that vulnerable populations such as Black SMM are not exploited. Additionally, sexual health prevention science might consider limiting fear-based or guilt-inducing messages that might cause unnecessary distress or stigmatization, especially among racial and sexual minority men. Ultimately, the ethical use of persuasion should build trust and support the overall well-being of individuals and communities.

Using In-Group Members as Public Health Interventionists

Chapters 3 and 6 respectively discussed the important and effective role of using in-group members to enhance study recruitment and serve as change agents in public health interventions among Black SMM. Some interventions (including POSSIBLE, Dangerfield II et al., 2024b, discussed in Chap. 7) recruit intervention staff from vulnerable communities based on their cultural similarities such as, race, sexual orientation, and community context, in addition to their health status to represent the interests of public health professionals (Kelly, 2004; Simoni et al., 2011; Weeks et al., 2009). The World Health Organization has also endorsed the use of community health workers, who are often members of target populations, to support public health organizations in marginalized communities (World Health Organization, 2018). However, using in-group members for health communication and public health interventions involves significant ethical considerations regarding the authenticity of the message and selecting individuals based upon race, sexuality, and health status. This approach also raises questions about fairness and exploitation because this can perpetuate stereotypes and reinforce stigmas within the community, as individuals are singled out for their health conditions rather than their contributions or capabilities. Using in-group members as interventionists could also suggest to the community that minority staff are only valued for their identity rather than their knowledge and contributions and inadvertently perpetuate stereotypes and reinforce existing stigmas (Dangerfield II & Wylie, 2022). Additionally, this other top-down approach could disrupt existing social dynamics and cohesion within the community because it could create divisions between public/community health workers and other community members (Dangerfield II, 2023). Although prevention scientists aim to enhance the credibility, relatability, and health literacy and benefits from the cultural similarity of peers, the broader social dynamics and the impact on community cohesion could be disregarded. My work suggests that some Black SMM do not want peers to replace clinicians because they do not want to abdicate healthcare providers from high standards of care (Dangerfield II et al., 2021a, 2022a). Therefore, it is crucial that prevention scientists carefully navigate these dynamics by ensuring that peer involvement complements (rather than substitutes) professional healthcare services and that in-group members are valued for their expertise, not just their identity.

Recruiting staff based on their health status or choosing representatives from vulnerable and marginalized communities can enhance the relatability and effectiveness of health messages. However, this approach must be handled with care to avoid tokenism, where individuals are chosen primarily for their minority status rather than their expertise or willingness. Ensuring that in-group members, peer change agents, or other representatives are genuinely engaged and empowered rather than being used as mere symbols is crucial to maintaining ethical integrity. Moreover, the potential impact on community interactions and networks cannot be ignored. Using in-group members without considering the broader social context and the long-term effects on community relationships can undermine trust and cooperation. Therefore, while leveraging in-group members can be an effective strategy for improving health interventions, it is essential to prioritize their well-being, provide ongoing support, and ensure that their involvement is part of a collaborative and respectful approach that benefits both the individuals and the community as a whole.

Targeting and Tailoring Public Health Messages

Chapter 7 described targeted and tailored public health messages involve health communication that established health-related goals in advance and then created messages that align with those objectives. Although targeted and tailored messages are essential and effective for effective health communication among minority communities, targeted and tailored health messages raise ethical concerns regarding exacerbating stigma to ensure the "common good." For example, when a campaign focuses exclusively on a particular demographic, such as Black gay men living with HIV, it can reinforce negative stereotypes and contribute to the perception that this group is uniquely problematic or at higher risk. The oversaturation of HIV-specific research and targeted interventions can increase prevention fatigue and concerns about further stigmatization among Black SMM (Arscott et al., 2019; Calabrese et al., 2023; Quinn et al., 2019). This can lead to further stigma, discrimination, and marginalization, exacerbating the very issues the campaign seeks to address. Additionally, segmenting and targeting certain groups inherently involves moral judgments regarding to equity and utility. Prioritizing "high risk" or "vulnerable" groups could lead to the exclusion of others who may be "hard to reach" and potentially marginalize these community members further. This selective approach can result in disparities where only certain segments benefit from health interventions, undermining the principle of equitable access to health resources.

To address the ethical challenges in targeted and tailored health communication for prevention research Black SMM, it is crucial that communicators first establish clear health-related goals and construct their messaging to align with objectives that align with the goals they have for themselves. This strategic approach ensures that all communications are purpose-driven and effective. Additionally, health communications should always aim to promote the "common good," a concept that must be defined through a community-driven standard, ensuring that the voices and needs of the community are at the forefront of intervention decision-making. When segmenting and targeting specific groups, such as Black SMM, communicators must navigate the moral judgments associated with equity and utility, striving to balance fairness and the greatest benefit for the most people. This approach not only respects the diverse experiences within the community but also promotes ethical integrity and trust in the research process.

Insufficient Informed Consent Details

Informed consent documents guide the basic ethical principles of human subjects research conduct as outlined by the Belmont Report (National Commission for the Protection of Human Subjects of Biomedical and Behavioral Research, 1979). The core tenets of the Belmont Report mandate that informed consent details the nature of the study, the benefits and risks involved in study participation, the randomization process (if applicable), and establishing participant comprehension prior to study enrollment. However, informed consent in research involving Black SMM faces unique challenges that highlight the need for culturally responsive approaches. Dome informed consent documents in sexual health prevention science might fail to include culturally relevant information despite existing protection guidelines. Specifically, Black SMM request that informed consent documents explicitly mention that researchers "will not hurt them" and that they "care for the overall health and wellness of Black gay men" (Dangerfield II et al., 2021a; Dangerfield II & Wylie, 2022). This is crucial because informed consent does involve knowledge of the study risks involved. However, these documents often lack the assurance and culturally specific language that would help build trust and reduce fears of exploitation or harm, which may not be possible. Including culturally relevant information and affirmations of care and respect in informed consent documents not only aligns with ethical research practices but also fosters a more inclusive and trustworthy environment for participants, ultimately enhancing the quality and effectiveness of the research. The ethical frameworks of justice and benefits within the Belmont Report may require more thoughtful considerations and specificity for this subpopulation when considering sexual health prevention science among Black SMM.

Randomization "Unfairness" and Therapeutic Misconception

Randomization is a fundamental process in clinical trial design in which participants are randomly assigned to different study groups, such as a treatment or control (placebo) group. Randomization ensures that each participant has an equal chance of being placed in any given group, which helps to eliminate selection bias and improves the credibility of the findings. It is a crucial component in maintaining the scientific rigor of clinical trials that lead to more accurate and credible conclusions about the efficacy and safety of new treatments or interventions. However, some young Black SMM in particular believe that randomization in prevention studies may not be fair for several reasons. One reason is that they believe that prevention scientists already assume (or know) that the experimental group is better than the standard of care (e.g., no intervention or minimal treatment) and to assign marginalized community members to a group that is hypothetically "worse" than the treatment group is unfair (Dangerfield II & Wylie, 2022). This is crucial to highlight because the assumption that one research group in a randomized controlled trial is more beneficial than the other undermines the presence of equipoise and raises questions regarding the ethical considerations of sexual health prevention science (Cook & Sheets, 2011; Dangerfield II & Wylie, 2022; McCambridge et al., 2014). Clinical equipoise means that there is no assumption on whether one treatment or intervention group is superior to another, justifying the need for a randomized trial to determine which is more effective. However, in sexual health prevention research, some randomized controlled trials are not necessarily investigated with equipoise; most have directional hypotheses intended to demonstrate the effectiveness of one intervention over another (Cook & Sheets, 2011; Gifford, 2001). Since contemporary randomized controlled trials intend to demonstrate some positive effect of the intervention compared to the standard of care, there are ethical considerations regarding equipoise that remain under discussed in HIV/STI prevention science. It is reasonable to anticipate that Black SMM would assume both that the treatment or experimental group is better than the control group and that the benefits of the treatment do not outweigh the effort involved in participation given their history of marginalization and minimal resources. Traditional designs of randomized controlled trials might not be culturally responsive to the needs of Black SMM and could perpetuate medical and research mistrust.

For traditionally low-resourced groups such as Black SMM, sexual health interventionists should reconsider study designs that have a group that receives "better treatment." Potentially, a single arm pre-test post-test interventional study could be more appropriate when the assumption is that the treatment is "better" than the standard of care, even though they are considered less rigorous than classic two-group randomized controlled trials. Studies should also request and secure additional funding and budget to accommodate the cultural responsive activities that may be required to engage with vulnerable population such as providing technological devices, transportation, and/or healthcare coverage for participants to sufficiently engage in the research (Dangerfield II & Wylie, 2022).

Typical Incentives as Inequitable

In Chap. 3, we discussed the crucial role of incentives in research and community engagement. Incentives promote fairness and ethical standards by acknowledging and valuing participants' time, effort, and contributions. Some Black gay men feel that typical incentives ($25–$50 cash or gift card) are inadequate and unfair for their participation, time, and effort reflecting a broader issue of undervaluation and exploitation within research practices. My studies have shown that Black SMM particularly advocate for incentives that help address their socio-economic needs and circumstances (Dangerfield II et al., 2018; Dangerfield II & Wylie, 2022).

Specifically, larger cash incentives (more than $50), transportation, healthcare coverage, and free experimental drugs are deemed as more relevant and equitable for their time, effort, and the potential risks or discomforts involved, given their unique cultural vulnerability (Dangerfield II et al., 2021b; White et al., 2019). These experiences is compounded by historical and ongoing mistrust in research institutions due to a legacy of exploitation and unethical practices in marginalized communities. Some also share that sexual health research participation is a mechanism for some low-resourced men to obtain medical or financial support via clinical care and cash incentives in prevention research. As a result, the perceived insufficiency of these incentives can deter their participation and retention, undermine trust, and hinder the recruitment of a diverse and representative sample, ultimately affecting the validity and inclusiveness of research findings.

There are no guidelines to help prevention scientists determine what "fair" incentives are for contemporary sexual health research, especially with Black SMM. There is also no consistency across Institutional Review Boards (IRB) and research sponsors on incentive what kinds of incentives are coercive. The primary purpose of an IRB is to protect the rights and welfare of human subjects. IRBs are responsible for reviewing research protocols and related materials to ensure that the methods used are ethical and that the potential benefits of the research justify any risks to participants. IRB policies and standards can vary significantly across institutions, leading to confusion and potential ethical dilemmas for scientists who aim to provide appropriate compensation without exerting undue influence. This lack of uniformity highlights the need for clear, culturally sensitive guidelines that address the unique challenges faced by researchers working with these vulnerable populations, ensuring ethical practices that promote both participation and equity in research. However, scientists must consider these perspectives and ensure that incentives are fair, equitable, and respectful of participants' contributions and lived experiences. Prevention scientists can ensure equitable and fair incentives for research participants by actively engaging with the communities they study to understand their needs, values, and perceptions of fair compensation. This involves conducting preliminary research or focus groups to gather input on what participants consider adequate and respectful compensation. Scientists can also collaborate with community leaders and advocacy groups to co-create incentive structures that are culturally sensitive and equitable. Scientists should also consider the socioeconomic backgrounds of participants and the potential burdens or risks associated with the study, adjusting incentives accordingly to ensure they reflect the true value of participants' time and contributions. Prevention scientists can foster greater participation, trust, and the overall success of their research endeavors by prioritizing fairness and actively addressing any concerns about undervaluation. Transparency is crucial; clearly communicating how incentive amounts are determined and ensuring they align with ethical guidelines helps build trust.

Harm Reduction Strategies

Harm reduction refers to practical strategies to minimize the negative health, social, and legal effects associated with certain high-risk behaviors, such as drug use. Harm reduction strategies seek to minimize the adverse health effects associated with risky behaviors without necessarily eliminating the behaviors themselves. Rather than focusing solely on abstinence, harm reduction acknowledges the reality of these behaviors and seeks to reduce their harmful consequences through evidence-based interventions (e.g., needle exchange or naloxone for overdose prevention). This pragmatic approach could clash with the ethical responsibility of health promotion and disease prevention and raise significant ethical concerns due to the delicate balance between reducing immediate risks and potentially endorsing or normalizing harmful behaviors. Harm reduction activities might implicitly condone illegal or dangerous activities and potentially undermine broader public health goals and societal norms. Ensuring that harm reduction messages are framed carefully to mitigate these ethical dilemmas while prioritizing the well-being and dignity of individuals remains a complex and ongoing challenge in prevention science and public health. Therefore, it is crucial to strike a balance that respects the complexities of harm reduction while steadfastly upholding the ethical imperatives of health promotion and disease prevention. This requires ongoing dialogue and collaboration among public health professionals, policymakers, and community stakeholders to ensure that harm reduction strategies do not inadvertently promote harmful behaviors but rather serve as a compassionate bridge towards healthier choices. Researchers can better address immediate risks while fostering long-term health and well-being for all individuals by carefully framing harm reduction messages and integrating them with broader public health initiatives.

Determining the Common Good

Determining the common good is necessary for ethical sexual health prevention science but presents some challenges when engaging with subpopulations. On one hand, we need standards that can be applied to all human subjects to promote uniformity and "fairness." On the other hand, targeted policies may be necessary to acknowledge specific cultural factors that might create differences in research understandings and participation. Therefore, prevention scientists can and should collaborate with community members to help build inclusivity, transparency, and trust. Community advisory boards or community panels can bringing together diverse groups of community members and harness a wide range of perspectives and experiences to inform decisions that affect impact the collective well-being. This participatory process not only ensures that the needs and values of the community are accurately reflected but also fosters trust, accountability, and a sense of responsibility towards the outcomes. Through open dialogue and mutual respect, community panels can effectively navigate complex issues and develop solutions that are equitable, sustainable, and genuinely beneficial for all members of society. To engage community members and improve ethical conduct in prevention science with Black SMM, consider the following community-based activities (Israel et al., 1998, 2010; White et al., 2019):

1. Collaborate with relevant experts and community representatives to identify health needs.
2. Determine suitable recommended responses to community health needs.
3. Prioritize community health needs and goals.
4. Engage interdisciplinary experts to design theoretically guided messages supporting the recommendations.
5. Design and test an ethical prevention strategy to effectively reach the target population.

Ethical Considerations for Engaging Community Advisory Boards

A community advisory board (CAB) is a group of community members who provide guidance, feedback, and support to researchers or organizations conducting projects within the community. CABs are essential in ensuring that the research or interventions are culturally sensitive, relevant, and ethically conducted. They help bridge the gap between the researchers and the community, fostering trust and cooperation. Ongoing community engagement and feedback are crucial for refining prevention strategies and ensuring they meet the needs of diverse populations. Collaborations between researchers, policymakers, and community leaders can enhance the effectiveness and acceptance of ethical prevention science. Although community advisory boards and other community panels can help improve ethical and equitable conduct, community members do not always understand clinical trial designs and could recommend approaches that could inadvertently affect the intervention's effects, necessitating clear communication and education from researchers. Additionally, community members often require personal investments of time and effort from prevention scientists and public health professionals, potentially challenging professional boundaries and necessitating careful navigation of these relationships. Compounding these issues is the lack of well-established guidelines for identifying equitable compensation for community members' contributions, which can lead to feelings of undervaluation and mistrust. Addressing these challenges requires a balanced approach that respects both the scientific integrity of the research and the valuable input and needs of the community.

Raised Questions

1. What ethical research mandates make research feel safe and equitable for Black SMM?
2. What informed consent details build trust and understanding to the satisfaction of Black SMM?
3. What are fair and equitable incentives for racial and sexual minority men's participation in prevention research studies?

Conclusion

Ethical prevention science conduct involves a commitment to upholding fundamental ethical principles throughout the research process, ensuring the protection and respect of all participants. This includes obtaining informed consent, ensuring confidentiality, protecting participant autonomy, and providing fair incentives as key components of respecting individuals' rights and maximizing benefits (Fisher, 2016). Researchers must obtain informed consent from participants, ensuring they are fully aware of the study's purpose, procedures, potential risks, and benefits. Ethical conduct also requires the avoidance of any form of bias or manipulation of data, ensuring that findings are reported accurately and without distortion. These ethical considerations are vital for maintaining public trust and promoting the development of effective and fair preventive interventions. No consensus has been established on ethical conduct across infectious and chronic disease health communication. Ethical domains must be considered in the planning and implementing of health communication programs and protocols. Collaborating with community members is key to improving ethical practice but also involves additional ethical/professional considerations, especially for marginalized minority communities. Future research should also test the relative impact of implementing these findings on research participation, acceptability, and trust among these racial and sexual minority men.

Chapter Summary

This chapter highlighted the importance of ethical research practices in prevention science, particularly with Black SMM, who have historically faced discrimination and marginalization. Ethical research conduct is crucial for ensuring the safety, integrity, and credibility of studies while promoting trust and equitable outcomes. The chapter discussed the application of ethical principles such as respect for persons, beneficence, and justice, and emphasizes the need for culturally tailored ethical frameworks that address the unique social, cultural, and emotional vulnerabilities of Black SMM. The chapter also addressed ethical challenges in using in-group members as public health interventionists, the impact of targeted health messages, informed consent insufficiencies, and the fairness of typical incentives. The chapter concluded by advocating for ongoing dialogue and adaptation of ethical guidelines to better serve marginalized communities.

Key Points

1. **Importance of ethical research conduct**: Black SMM often approach research with caution, necessitating a focus on building trust and ensuring ethical conduct, especially in sexual health prevention science. Ethical research conduct is crucial for maintaining integrity, protecting participants, and ensuring credible, socially responsible science. Key ethical principles outlined by the Belmont Report—respect for persons, beneficence, and justice—guide researchers in obtaining informed consent, minimizing harm, and ensuring equitable treatment of participants, especially within marginalized communities like Black SMM.
2. **Culturally responsive ethical frameworks**: Ethical guidelines must be tailored to address the unique social, cultural, and emotional vulnerabilities of Black SMM, ensuring trust and meaningful participation in research.
3. **Persuasive communication tactics**: Health promotion strategies must balance effective messaging with respect for autonomy and avoid manipulative tactics that could undermine the trust and freedom of participants.
4. **Informed consent and randomization concerns**: Black SMM often feel that informed consent documents lack culturally relevant information, such as assurances that researchers care about their well-being. Additionally, some Black SMM perceive randomization in clinical trials as unfair, especially when they believe one group is receiving a superior intervention. These concerns highlight the need for more culturally responsive consent processes and reconsideration of study designs to build trust and address issues of fairness
5. **Ethical use of in-group members as interventionists**: Using in-group members (e.g., peers from the same racial or sexual minority) as interventionists can enhance intervention relatability and effectiveness, but it also raises ethical concerns. These include potential tokenism, reinforcing stereotypes, and creating divisions within the community. Care must be taken to ensure that in-group members are valued for their expertise and that their involvement complements professional healthcare services rather than replacing them.
6. **Fair incentives**: Many Black SMM feel that typical research incentives are inadequate and do not reflect the value of their participation, particularly given their socioeconomic challenges. There are no consistent guidelines across Institutional Review Boards (IRBs) on what constitutes fair compensation. Researchers must ensure that incentives are fair, equitable, and sensitive to the lived experiences of participants to foster trust and participation.

References

Arnold, E. A., Rebchook, G. M., & Kegeles, S. M. (2014). "Triply cursed": Racism, homophobia, and HIV-related stigma are barriers to regular HIV testing, treatment adherence, and disclosure among young Black gay men. *Culture, Health & Sexuality, 16*(6), 710–722. https://doi.org/10.1080/13691058.2014.905706

Arrington-Sanders, R., Hailey-Fair, K., Wirtz, A. L., Morgan, A., Brooks, D., Castillo, M., Trexler, C., Kwait, J., Dowshen, N., Galai, N., Beyrer, C., & Celentano, D. (2020). Role of structural marginalization, HIV stigma, and mistrust on HIV prevention and treatment among young Black Latinx men who have sex with men and transgender women: Perspectives from youth service providers. *AIDS Patient Care and STDs, 34*(1), 7–15. https://doi.org/10.1089/apc.2019.0165

Arscott, J., Humphreys, J., Merwin, E., & Relf, M. (2019). "That Guy is Gay and Black. That's a Red Flag." How HIV stigma and racism affect perception of risk among young Black men who have sex with men. *AIDS and Behavior, 24*, 173–184. https://doi.org/10.1007/s10461-019-02607-4

Cahill, S., Taylor, S. W., Elsesser, S. A., Mena, L., Hickson, D., & Mayer, K. H. (2017). Stigma, medical mistrust, and perceived racism may affect PrEP awareness and uptake in black compared to white gay and bisexual men in Jackson, Mississippi and Boston, Massachusetts. *AIDS Care, 29*(11), 1351–1358. https://doi.org/10.1080/09540121.2017.1300633

Calabrese, S. K., Kalwicz, D. A., Dovidio, J. F., Rao, S., Modrakovic, D. X., Boone, C. A., Magnus, M., Kharfen, M., Patel, V. V., & Zea, M. C. (2023). Targeted social marketing of PrEP and the stigmatization of Black sexual minority men. *PLoS One, 18*(5), e0285329. https://doi.org/10.1371/journal.pone.0285329

Cook, C., & Sheets, C. (2011). Clinical equipoise and personal equipoise: Two necessary ingredients for reducing bias in manual therapy trials. *The Journal of Manual & Manipulative Therapy, 19*(1), 55–57. https://doi.org/10.1179/106698111X12899036752014

Dangerfield, D. T., II. (2023). A principal investigator as a PrEP-using peer change agent for HIV prevention among Black gay and bisexual men: An autoethnography. *International Journal of Environmental Research and Public Health, 20*(7), 5309. https://doi.org/10.3390/ijerph20075309

Dangerfield, D. T., II, & Wylie, C. (2022). Identifying ethical and culturally responsive research activities to build trust and improve participation of Black sexual minority men in pre-exposure prophylaxis telehealth clinical trials: Qualitative study. *JMIR Human Factors, 9*(1), e28798. https://doi.org/10.2196/28798

Dangerfield, D. T., II, Harawa, N. T., McWells, C., Hilliard, C., & Bluthenthal, R. N. (2018). Exploring the preferences of a culturally congruent, peer-based HIV prevention intervention for Black men who have sex with men. *Sexual Health, 15*(5), 424–430. https://doi.org/10.1071/SH18057

Dangerfield, D. T., II, Cooper, J., Heidari, O., Allen, S., Winder, T. J. A., & Lucas, G. M. (2021a). Nursing and health care preferences among opioid and stimulant using Black sexual minority men: An exploratory study. *Journal of the Association of Nurses in AIDS Care, 32*(5), e30–e39. https://doi.org/10.1097/JNC.0000000000000201

Dangerfield, D. T., II, Wylie, C., & Anderson, J. N. (2021b). Conducting virtual, synchronous focus groups among Black sexual minority men: Qualitative study. *JMIR Public Health and Surveillance, 7*(2), e22980. https://doi.org/10.2196/22980

Dangerfield, D. T., II, Lipson, A., & Anderson, J. N. (2022a). HIV PrEP clinician communication preferences among Black sexual minority men. *AIDS Education and Prevention, 34*(2), 168–181. https://doi.org/10.1521/aeap.2022.34.2.168

Dangerfield, D. T., II, Anderson, J. N., Wylie, C., Arrington-Sanders, R., Bluthenthal, R. N., Beyrer, C., & Farley, J. E. (2022b). Refining a multicomponent intervention to increase perceived HIV risk and PrEP initiation: Focus group study among Black sexual minority men. *JMIR Formative Research, 6*(8), e34181. https://doi.org/10.2196/34181

Dangerfield, D. T., II, Anderson, J. N., & Tinnell, T. (2024a). Cultural acceptability of STI screening guidelines and sexual positioning assessments among Black sexual minority men. *Journal of Advanced Nursing, 80*(8), 3253–3263. https://doi.org/10.1111/jan.16017

Dangerfield, D. T., II, Anderson, J. N., Wylie, C., Bluthenthal, R., Beyrer, C., & Farley, J. E. (2024b). A multicomponent intervention (POSSIBLE) to improve perceived risk for HIV among Black sexual minority men: Feasibility and preliminary effectiveness pilot study. *JMIR Human Factors, 11*(1), e54739. https://doi.org/10.2196/54739

Fisher, C. B. (2016). *Decoding the ethics code: A practical guide for psychologists*. Sage.

Gifford, F. (2001). Uncertainty about clinical equipoise. *BMJ: British Medical Journal, 322*(7289), 795.

Israel, M., & Hay, I. (2006). *Research ethics for social scientists*. Sage.

Israel, B. A., Schulz, A. J., Parker, E. A., & Becker, A. B. (1998). Review of community-based research: Assessing partnership approaches to improve public health. *Annual Review of Public Health, 19*(1), 173–202. https://doi.org/10.1146/annurev.publhealth.19.1.173

Israel, B. A., Coombe, C. M., Cheezum, R. R., Schulz, A. J., McGranaghan, R. J., Lichtenstein, R., Reyes, A. G., Clement, J., & Burris, A. (2010). Community-based participatory research: A capacity-building approach for policy advocacy aimed at eliminating health disparities. *American Journal of Public Health, 100*(11), 2094–2102. https://doi.org/10.2105/AJPH.2009.170506

Jacobs, N. (2020). Two ethical concerns about the use of persuasive technology for vulnerable people. *Bioethics, 34*(5), 519–526. https://doi.org/10.1111/bioe.12683

Kelly, J. A. (2004). Popular opinion leaders and HIV prevention peer education: Resolving discrepant findings, and implications for the development of effective community programmes. *AIDS Care, 16*(2), 139–150. https://doi.org/10.1080/09540120410001640986

McCambridge, J., Kypri, K., & Elbourne, D. (2014). In randomization we trust? There are overlooked problems in experimenting with people in behavioral intervention trials. *Journal of Clinical Epidemiology, 67*(3), 247–253. https://doi.org/10.1016/j.jclinepi.2013.09.004

Moravcsik, A. (2019). *Transparency in qualitative research*. Sage. https://doi.org/10.4135/9781526421036

National Commission for the Protection of Human Subjects of Biomedical and Behavioral Research. (1979). *The Belmont Report*. https://www.hhs.gov/ohrp/regulations-and-policy/belmont-report/read-the-belmont-report/index.html

Parrott, R. (2008). A multiple discourse approach to health communication: Translational research and ethical practice. *Journal of Applied Communication Research, 36*(1), 1–7. https://doi.org/10.1080/00909880701799345

Quinn, K., Bowleg, L., & Dickson-Gomez, J. (2019). "The fear of being Black plus the fear of being gay": The effects of intersectional stigma on PrEP use among young Black gay, bisexual, and other men who have sex with men. *Social Science & Medicine, 232*, 86–93. https://doi.org/10.1016/j.socscimed.2019.04.042

Rosenstock, I. M. (1974). Historical origins of the health belief model. *Health Education Monographs, 2*(4), 328–335. https://doi.org/10.1177/109019817400200403

Rossi, J., & Yudell, M. (2012). The use of persuasion in public health communication: An ethical critique. *Public Health Ethics, 5*(2), 192–205. https://doi.org/10.1093/phe/phs019

Scharff, D. P., Mathews, K. J., Jackson, P., Hoffsuemmer, J., Martin, E., & Edwards, D. (2010). More than Tuskegee: Understanding mistrust about research participation. *Journal of Health Care for the Poor and Underserved, 21*(3), 879–897. https://doi.org/10.1353/hpu.0.0323

Simoni, J. M., Nelson, K. M., Franks, J. C., Yard, S. S., & Lehavot, K. (2011). Are peer interventions for HIV efficacious? A systematic review. *AIDS and Behavior, 15*(8), 1589–1595. https://doi.org/10.1007/s10461-011-9963-5

Weeks, M. R., Convey, M., Dickson-Gomez, J., Li, J., Radda, K., Martinez, M., & Robles, E. (2009). Changing drug users' risk environments: Peer health advocates as multi-level community change agents. *American Journal of Community Psychology, 43*(3), 330–344. https://doi.org/10.1007/s10464-009-9234-z

White, J. J., Dangerfield, D. T., II, & Grieb, S. M. (2019). Methodological considerations for conducting focus groups in HIV prevention research among Black men who have sex with men. *Public Health Nursing, 36*(3), 439–445. https://doi.org/10.1111/phn.12592

Witte, K. (1992). Putting the fear back into fear appeals: The extended parallel process model. *Communication Monographs, 59*(4), 329–349. https://doi.org/10.1080/03637759209376276

World Health Organization. (2017). *Code of conduct for responsible research.* World Health Organization. https://cdn.who.int/media/docs/default-source/wpro%2D%2D-documents/regional-committee/nomination-regional-director/code-of-conduct/ccrr.pdf?sfvrsn=b2cb450_2&ua=1

World Health Organization. (2018). *WHO guideline on health policy and system support to optimize community health worker programmes.* World Health Organization. https://iris.who.int/handle/10665/275474

Chapter 10
Next Steps for Sexual Health Prevention Science and Methods with Black SMM

Next Steps

As this handbook comes to a close, the conclusions presented encapsulate key insights from over a decade of research focused on advancing sexual health prevention for Black gay, bisexual, and other Black SMM in light of the current scientific, epidemiological, and cultural landscape. This body of work underscores the urgent need for contemporary, targeted (yet sensitive), culturally responsive methods that address the unique challenges faced by this community. Persistent barriers such as health beliefs, medical mistrust, and social inequalities contribute to the ongoing disparities in HIV/STI outcomes among Black SMM. This handbook empowers prevention scientists, clinicians, and public health practitioners to refine and elevate their approaches using mindful and relevant scientific methods, culturally responsive interventions, and ethical research practices. The conclusions drawn from this work not only reflect the current state of sexual health prevention science but also lay the foundation for future research, interventions, and strategies for the community.

Focus on Sexual Epidemiology

Prevention science should prioritize and build upon the field of sexual epidemiology to better understand the complex factors driving HIV and STI outcomes. The underexplored role of sexual positioning among SMM generally and Black SMM specifically and whether individuals identify as tops, bottoms, versatile, or something else significantly influences same-sex dynamics. Yet these behavioral and cultural dynamics remain insufficiently addressed in current sexual health prevention science studies. The field of sexual epidemiology can provide key insights into the

D. T. Dangerfield II, *Prevention Science & Targeted Methods for HIV/STI Research with Black Sexual Minority Men*,
https://doi.org/10.1007/978-3-031-85130-8_10

HIV/STI related outcomes but is still in its nascent stages. Longitudinal studies should be conducted to explore how sexual positioning, role identities, and behaviors evolve over time and how these changes impact health outcomes. Adapting public health interventions to account for these variations in sexual roles and behaviors can enhance their effectiveness, ensuring that prevention strategies are relevant and responsive to the specific needs of Black SMM. To sufficiently understand the lifestyles, risks, and sexual health vulnerabilities of Black SMM, studies must be grounded in an understanding of the socio-cultural dynamics that shape sexual behaviors and health outcomes within this population. This also includes recognizing and addressing the stigma, discrimination, and medical mistrust that often create barriers to accessing healthcare and prevention resources, which are impacted by sexuality. Prevention science and public health practitioners can become more inclusive of and effective for Black SMM by integrating nuanced sexual epidemiology with other culturally responsive approaches.

Contemporary Recruitment and Engagement Methods

Post-COVID-19, digital platforms have emerged as crucial tools for research and community engagement across populations. However, the underutilization of targeted digital health strategies among Black SMM indicates a missed opportunity to connect with this community through innovative and accessible means. Digital strategies must engage Black SMM in research and healthcare, especially in light of prevalent medical and research mistrust. These strategies should be designed to meet the community where they are, using technology that is accessible, user-friendly, and private. Online platforms, mobile apps, and virtual counseling sessions provide accessible and flexible options for delivering health education and support and can offer interactive content, personalized feedback, and real-time communication with clinicians/interventionists for easier access and support. Incorporating technology and digital health innovations can also significantly enhance sexual health prevention for Black SMM. Technological innovations such as telehealth, artificial intelligence (AI), and big data can offer new tools and approaches to overcome existing barriers and improve health outcomes on a broader scale. Mobile health applications, telehealth services, and online educational platforms can provide accessible and confidential resources for Black SMM. The expansion of telemedicine services offers a promising avenue for enhancing HIV prevention and care, particularly for Black SMM who face barriers to accessing traditional healthcare settings. This is especially beneficial in reducing stigma and increasing accessibility for those living in rural or underserved areas. mHealth apps are another technological innovation transforming HIV prevention. Apps tailored to the needs of Black SMM can provide culturally relevant content and support, enhancing their engagement with prevention strategies by offering a range of services, including reminders for medication adherence, educational resources, risk assessment tools, and direct communication with clinicians.

Scaling Person-Centered Statistical Approaches

Scaling person-centered statistical approaches in HIV/STI prevention science is crucial for desinging more effective and targeted health interventions. Big data analytics and AI have the potential to revolutionize how prevention scientists and clinicians track, predict, and respond to disease patterns by analyzing vast datasets from sources such as social media, public health records, electronic health records, and social determinants of health. These technologies can identify emerging trends and high-risk areas for outbreaks, enabling the rapid deployment of resources and the development of tailored interventions that directly address the needs of the most vulnerable individuals For example, predictive analyses can help clinicians prioritize resources by pinpointing individuals who may benefit the most from targeted prevention efforts, improving overall efficacy and outcomes. In addition to enhancing resource allocation, the use of advanced data analytics and AI can personalize health interventions, making them more responsive to individual behaviors, preferences, and health conditions. Machine learning algorithms can analyze individual-level data to design interventions that are specifically tailored to meet the unique needs of each person. Scaling these person-centered approaches will not only enhance the precision of interventions but could also foster greater engagement and trust, ultimately reducing health disparities and improving sexual health outcomes in the community.

Leveraging Qualitative Methods for Research and Intervention Design

Qualitative methods delve into the experiences, attitudes, perceptions, and cultural contexts that shape health behaviors. These in-depth insights are crucial for understanding the unique challenges that Black SMM face, including navigating stigma, discrimination, and resource instability. To maximize the impact of prevention science, it is important to prioritize ongoing qualitative research that continues to explore the diverse and evolving experiences of Black SMM. This research should not only inform intervention design but also guide the development of communication strategies, policy advocacy, and community engagement efforts that resonate with Black SMM. This approach allows for the creation of interventions that are more likely to be accepted and adopted by the community because they reflect their values, concerns, and lived realities. Moreover, qualitative research can help identify gaps in existing interventions, providing a feedback loop that enables continuous refinement and adaptation of strategies as new insights emerge. Prioritizing qualitative research can help prevention scientists and public health professionals create more holistic and impactful interventions that address the complex social, cultural, and psychological factors influencing the sexual health of Black SMM. This commitment to understanding and valuing the voices of Black SMM will ultimately lead to more effective, equitable, and sustainable health outcomes.

Scaling Peer-Based Interventions

Peer-led interventions are and will likely continue to be highly effective in promoting health behaviors and providing support for Black SMM. To diffuse and maximize the impact of novel and effective biomedical and behavioral interventions for Black SMM, it is crucial to address barriers to access, uptake, and adherence: stigma, lack of awareness, risk perceptions, healthcare access, and socioeconomic factors. Interventions must be designed to educate communities, reduce stigma, and provide support systems that facilitate easier access to and consistent use of prevention regimens (behavioral and biomedical). Community-based programs that leverage peer change agents (PCAs) who can relate to and effectively communicate with others are promising for sexual health promotion. These approaches leverage the deep understanding peers have of cultural and social contexts. Expanding the use of peer change agents in sexual health interventions, leveraging their unique positions within the community to address stigma, promote safer sex practices, and facilitate the uptake of preventive measures like PrEP. These interventions often combine communication strategies such as motivational interviewing with other approaches such as technology to create a supportive environment for behavior change. Strengthening behavioral interventions should involve training peers to deliver accurate health information, provide emotional support, and serve as role models. Integrating sexual role considerations into the development of peer-led interventions can further enhance their effectiveness. PCAs who share similar sexual role experiences with the target population can serve as credible sources of information and support, helping to normalize discussions around sexual positioning and reduce associated stigma. By addressing the multifaceted barriers through culturally competent and community-driven approaches, prevention science can improve PrEP uptake and adherence, ultimately reducing HIV/STI transmission rates and promoting overall sexual health among Black SMM. These efforts should also be supported by ongoing research to identify and address gaps in knowledge and implementation, ensuring that interventions remain relevant and responsive to the evolving needs of the community. Additionally, integrating digital health tools and telehealth platforms into these interventions can further expand access and reduce logistical barriers. Combining culturally tailored education, peer-led initiatives, policy advocacy, and technological innovation can create a comprehensive and sustainable framework for reducing health disparities and improving the sexual health outcomes of Black SMM.

Implementing Targeted and Tailored Interventions

Contemporary behavioral HIV/STI prevention interventions have evolved from simplistic, single-focus strategies to more comprehensive, multicomponent approaches. These modern interventions must address the social, psychological, and structural barriers that Black SMM encounter, such as stigma, discrimination, healthcare access, and socioeconomic inequalities. Implementing targeted and tailored sexual health interventions for Black SMM must be designed with an acute awareness of the specific needs, challenges, and cultural contexts of Black SMM, which will help to reduce the significant health disparities they face. By focusing on tailored strategies that promote safer sexual practices and expand access to preventive measures like PrEP, public health efforts can become more effective in addressing the complex factors that influence sexual health behaviors in this population. By investing in the development and rigorous testing of sexual health interventions tailored to the diverse subgroups within the Black SMM community—such as those in the house/ballroom scene, leather communities, and other distinct cultural groups—public health initiatives can ensure that these efforts are both widely applicable and effective in reducing health disparities. Moreover, public health campaigns should leverage social marketing strategies that resonate with the lived experiences of Black SMM, using culturally relevant messaging to reduce stigma and increase awareness about prevention options. These campaigns must be sensitive to the unique social dynamics and communication preferences within the community to foster greater engagement and acceptance.

In designing targeted and tailored sexual health interventions, it is essential to consider the diverse sexual roles—such as tops, bottoms, and versatile individuals—that play a significant yet often underexplored role in shaping sexual health behaviors and outcomes. These roles not only influence risk perceptions but also affect HIV/STI transmission dynamics, making it crucial to tailor interventions accordingly. Public health strategies that acknowledge and address the specific concerns, behaviors, and vulnerabilities associated with different sexual roles can greatly enhance the effectiveness of prevention efforts. Interventions must account for the fluidity and complexity of sexual role identities, recognizing that individuals may not always adhere strictly to their self-identified roles. This understanding can help in crafting more nuanced and responsive interventions that provide tailored, stigma-free support across various sexual behaviors. For instance, prevention messages and counseling should be adaptable to the needs of tops, bottoms, and versatile individuals, offering role-specific information about risk reduction strategies, such as PrEP use, condom negotiation, and regular testing.

Addressing Sexual Health Misinformation and Mistrust

Reducing misinformation and medical mistrust among Black SMM requires a multi-faceted approach in which researchers and clinicians play crucial roles. Building trust between these professionals and the community is critical for ensuring that accurate sexual health information is accepted and acted upon. To do this, clinicians and researchers must adopt culturally competent approaches that prioritize open communication, respect, and empathy. These professionals should be trained to recognize and address the historical and ongoing factors that contribute to medical mistrust, such as discrimination, stigma, and the legacy of unethical research practices targeting Black communities. By acknowledging these factors, they can create a more supportive and trusting environment for Black SMM.

Researchers can also contribute to reducing misinformation by designing studies that are transparent, community-centered, and ethically sound. Involving Black SMM in the research process from the outset—through participatory research models or community advisory boards—ensures that the research is relevant and that findings are communicated in ways that resonate with the community. Additionally, researchers should prioritize the dissemination of their findings to the community in accessible formats, ensuring that the results of studies are not just published in academic journals but also shared with the populations they aim to serve. This practice of returning results to the community can enhance transparency, build trust, and directly address any misconceptions that may arise from the research process. Clinicians, in particular, are in a unique position to counter misinformation during routine healthcare visits. They can provide patients with accurate, up-to-date information on sexual health topics such as HIV prevention, PrEP, and STI testing. However, delivering this information effectively requires sensitivity to the cultural and social contexts of Black SMM. Clinicians should engage in conversations that validate the patient's experiences and concerns, using language that is inclusive and non-judgmental. Building rapport, demonstrating genuine care, and staying updated with the prevention science landscape can establish clinicians as trusted sources of information, thereby reducing the influence of misinformation.

Researchers and clinicians can work together to develop and implement community outreach programs that focus on education and engagement. These programs can be designed to provide accurate health information while also addressing the root causes of medical mistrust. Collaborations with trusted community leaders and organizations can enhance the credibility of these efforts, ensuring that messages are more likely to be received and trusted by Black SMM. Creating spaces for dialogue and providing consistent, evidence-based information can help clinicians and researchers gradually chip away at the misinformation and mistrust that have long hindered progress in sexual health prevention for this community.

Revisiting Research Ethics

Ensuring ethical conduct in HIV prevention research is paramount to building trust, fostering participation, and ultimately improving health outcomes with Black SMM. Ethical considerations must prioritize the protection and respect of participants through informed consent, confidentiality, and autonomy, while also ensuring that the research provides tangible benefits to the community. Given the history of medical exploitation and ongoing disparities in healthcare access, addressing medical mistrust within this population is crucial. Researchers must engage with Black SMM communities in a transparent and culturally sensitive manner, ensuring that the research is both respectful and aligned with the community's needs. This involves fostering collaborative relationships with community leaders and organizations, which can serve as trusted intermediaries in the research process. Additionally, fair and timely incentives, clear communication of research goals, and the assurance of privacy are essential to mitigate skepticism and enhance participation. Next steps in ethical research must standardize of ethical guidelines that prioritize the protection of Black SMM in all phases of research, from study design to dissemination of results. Researchers should also consider creating participatory research models that actively involve Black SMM in the decision-making process, ensuring that their voices are heard and that the research directly addresses their needs and concerns. Ethical considerations must also extend to the implementation of research findings, ensuring that interventions are not only effective but also equitable and accessible.

Addressing Socioecological Barriers

Addressing the social determinants of health—such as housing, employment, health literacy, and healthcare access—is essential for improving the sexual health outcomes of Black SMM. Expanding access to healthcare is a crucial step, particularly by increasing the availability of HIV/STI testing, prevention, and treatment services in underserved areas through mobile clinics, telehealth, and community health centers. Policies that promote healthcare coverage, like Medicaid expansion, are necessary to ensure that more people have access to essential services. Beyond healthcare, policies must address socioeconomic disparities by fostering economic stability and access to quality education, which support healthier lifestyles and reduce HIV transmission rates. Integrating social services with health interventions is vital for tackling the root causes of the observed population differences in sexual health outcomes. Additionally, addressing structural barriers such as racism, discrimination, and stigma remains a priority. Expanding healthcare access, enforcing anti-discrimination laws, and providing economic support are crucial for improving health outcomes. Legal protections that reduce stigma and discrimination—such as equal rights laws, protections against discrimination, and recognition of same-sex partnerships—can significantly affect both the mental and physical health of Black SMM. Public awareness campaigns and education programs that promote acceptance of sexual minorities further reduce societal stigma, helping to create inclusive communities where individuals feel valued and cared for, which is critical for their overall health and quality of life.

More Black Gay Scientists

Research consistently indicates that Black SMM prefer and respond more positively to sexual health interventions led by Black/gay scientists (Dangerfield et al., 2022; Dangerfield II & Wylie, 2022). Data from the Pew Research Center also showed that Black Americans are more likely to engage in science and medicine when they see successful Black people in the field (Funk, 2022). Generally, investigators from target populations enhance research designs, validity, and participant engagement because they have insider perspectives and can build trust and address community-specific needs effectively. Black SMM might perceive Black/gay-led research teams as more culturally sensitive, trustworthy, and capable of understanding their unique socioecological challenges, such as racism, homophobia, and trauma than others. Therefore, Black gay scientists are needed to build trust, identify relevant measures and approaches for studies, and improve clinical engagement among Black SMM. Having research teams reflects the target population's cultural background and experiences could foster a greater sense of representation and safety, which is crucial for the success of community-centered interventions. This alignment could not only improves recruitment and retention but also ensures that the findings and interventions are more relevant and effective. The field can make significant strides in reducing disparities and promoting health equity for Black SMM communities by increasing the number of Black gay scientists and integrating their expertise into sexual health research.

Training and Education for Clinicians

Patient-clinician communication remains a substantial barrier for optimal sexual health among Black SMM. There is a significant gap in culturally competent approaches to sexual health care for Black SMM, resulting in medical mistrust and low treatment adherence. Researchers and clinicians often fail to understand or address the unique needs of this community, which hinders their engagement and retention in research and clinical care. Clinicians require comprehensive training in the health needs of racial and sexual minorities to effectively prevent HIV and STIs. By incorporating education on the specific sexual health needs and behaviors of racial and sexual minorities into clinical curricula, clinicians can better understand and address the unique risks and barriers faced by Black SMM. Training clinicians and health educators key issues in the behavioral, social, and cultural dynamics of Black SMM can also improve their ability to deliver information in a way that is respectful and responsive to the needs of the community. This can involve incorporating culturally relevant examples, language, and visuals, as well as addressing specific cultural beliefs and practices. This and other forms of training is crucial for addressing the unique barriers Black SMM populations face, including stigma, prejudice, and misinformation that can hinder access to care and adherence to prevention strategies. Enhanced training programs can equip healthcare professionals with the skills to create more inclusive and supportive environments. Invest in training for healthcare providers and researchers to improve cultural competency and sensitivity when working with Black SMM. This includes developing curricula that address the unique sexual health needs and experiences of this community.

Conclusion

The future of sexual health prevention science with Black SMM hinges on the integration of contemporary methodologies, interdisciplinary collaboration, and a deep commitment to cultural responsiveness. Addressing the complex needs of this community requires intentionality, methodological transparency, and consistent efforts to understand the population and build trust. Although existing qualitative and quantitative research methods must be adapted to be more culturally responsive, there is also a pressing need to innovate new methods that better capture the diverse experiences and health behaviors of Black SMM. Prevention science can make significant strides toward reducing negative sexual health outcomes in the community through ethical, consistent, and culturally attuned research practices. Equally important is the commitment to continuous evaluation and adaptation of interventions. Health behaviors and social contexts are dynamic, and prevention strategies must be regularly reassessed and refined in light of emerging evidence and community feedback. This iterative process is essential to ensure that interventions remain effective, relevant, and capable of addressing the evolving needs of Black SMM. Ultimately, by advancing these strategies, sexual health prevention science can foster more equitable and impactful health outcomes, reduce STI/HIV transmission, and improve the overall quality of life among Black SMM.

References

Dangerfield, D., II, & Wylie, C. (2022). Identifying ethical and culturally responsive research activities to build trust and improve participation of black sexual minority men in pre-exposure prophylaxis telehealth clinical trials: Qualitative study. *JMIR Human Factors, 9*(1), e28798. https://doi.org/10.2196/28798

Dangerfield, D. T., II, Lipson, A., & Anderson, J. N. (2022). HIV PrEP clinician communication preferences among black sexual minority men. *AIDS Education and Prevention, 34*(2), 168–181. https://doi.org/10.1521/aeap.2022.34.2.168

Funk, C. (2022, April 7). *Black Americans' views of and engagement with science.* Pew Research Center. https://www.pewresearch.org/science/2022/04/07/black-americans-views-of-and-engagement-with-science/

MIX
Papier aus verantwortungsvollen Quellen
Paper from responsible sources
FSC® C105338

If you have any concerns about our products,
you can contact us on
ProductSafety@springernature.com

In case Publisher is established outside the EU,
the EU authorized representative is:
Springer Nature Customer Service Center GmbH
Europaplatz 3, 69115 Heidelberg, Germany

Printed by Libri Plureos GmbH
in Hamburg, Germany